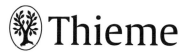

Atlas of Injection
Therapy in Pain Management

Juergen Fischer, MD

Professor
Specialist in Orthopedics and Trauma Surgery
Orthopedic Center Luisenplatz
Darmstadt, Germany

95 illustrations

Thieme
Stuttgart · New York

Library of Congress Cataloging-in-Publication Data

Fischer, Jürgen, MD.
  [Schmerztherapie mit Lokalanästethika. English]
  Atlas of injection therapy in pain management : injection techniques simple and safe / Juergen Fischer.
     p. ; cm.
  Includes bibliographical references and index.
  ISBN 978-3-13-154301-1 (alk. paper)
  1.Injections, Intra-articular–Atlases. 2.Joints–Diseases–Chemotherapy–Atlases. I. Title.
  [DNLM: 1.Pain–drug therapy–Atlases. 2.Anesthetics, Local–therapeutic use–Atlases. 3.Injections–methods–Atlases. WL 17]
  RC925.5.F57 2011
  616'.0472–dc23
                                   2011018960

This book is an authorized translation of the 2nd German edition published and copyrighted 2010 by Georg Thieme Verlag, Stuttgart. Title of the German edition: Schmerztherapie mit Lokalanästhetika. Injektionstechniken – einfach und sicher.

Translator: Ruth Gutberlet, Cochem, Germany

Illustrator: Christine Lackner, Ittlingen; Peter Haller, Stuttgart; Holger Vanselow, Stuttgart, Germany

© 2012 Georg Thieme Verlag,
Rüdigerstrasse 14, 70469 Stuttgart, Germany
http://www.thieme.de
Thieme New York, 333 Seventh Avenue,
New York, NY 10001, USA
http://www.thieme.com

Cover design: Thieme Publishing Group
Typesetting by SOMMER media GmbH & Co. KG,
Feuchtwangen, Germany
Printed in China by Everbest Printing Co, Ltd.

ISBN 978-3-13-154301-1   1 2 3 4 5 6

Important note: Medicine is an ever-changing science undergoing continual development. Research and clinical experience are continually expanding our knowledge, in particular our knowledge of proper treatment and drug therapy. Insofar as this book mentions any dosage or application, readers may rest assured that the authors, editors, and publishers have made every effort to ensure that such references are in accordance with **the state of knowledge at the time of production of the book.**

Nevertheless, this does not involve, imply, or express any guarantee or responsibility on the part of the publishers in respect to any dosage instructions and forms of applications stated in the book. **Every user is requested to examine carefully** the manufacturers' leaflets accompanying each drug and to check, if necessary in consultation with a physician or specialist, whether the dosage schedules mentioned therein or the contraindications stated by the manufacturers differ from the statements made in the present book. Such examination is particularly important with drugs that are either rarely used or have been newly released on the market. Every dosage schedule or every form of application used is entirely at the user's own risk and responsibility. The authors and publishers request every user to report to the publishers any discrepancies or inaccuracies noticed. If errors in this work are found after publication, errata will be posted at www.thieme.com on the product description page.

Dedicated to my children
Kai and Nicole

Preface

Pain is the most frequent cause for patient–physician contact. The patient expects rapid relief and freedom from pain. The more efficient the relief, the more successful the physician is felt to be.

Besides elimination of pain-producing causes, elimination of pain itself is the ultimate ambition of therapy. This should take place rapidly, with few side effects, simply, and at little cost.

Pain treatment through local anesthetics is one of the most efficient and fastest-acting pain treatment options. A prerequisite is knowledge of the exact techniques and indications, as well as the risks. Injections are invasive procedures and require precise execution. Pain symptoms and patterns encountered in daily practice are manifold and often difficult to associate causally. Among the various pain patterns that present themselves in daily practice, some typical, constantly recurring patterns emerge. The typical clinical pain pattern allows exact assignment of a suitable injection treatment.

In this book, physicians will find symptom-oriented "cookbook-style" directions, which provide easy recognition and indication of the approach. Both circumscribed pain of singular origin and complex pain syndromes can be managed effectively and rapidly.

Owing to the great number of didactical illustrations, it is possible to perform injection treatments with little preceding experience. Risks are discernable in regard to technique and location and concomitant treatments are listed. This enables the practitioner to rid the patient of pain in a fast, efficient, and low-risk manner.

Juergen Fischer

Contents

5 Thorax and Abdomen

6 Lumbar Spine and Pelvis

7 Lower Extremities

Abbreviations

Acu	acupuncture/acupressure
Auto	autogenic training
BFB	biofeedback therapy
Chiro	chiropractic treatment
Cryo	cryotherapy
ENT	otolaryngological medicine (ear, nose, throat)
ESWL	extracorporeal shock wave lithotripsy
FMA	friction massage
Gen	general medical treatment
Gyn	gynecological treatment
Int	internal medicine therapy
MA	massages
Med	medication
MET	medical exercise therapy
MM	manual mobilization
MR	muscular relaxation techniques, for example, the Jacobson technique
Nut	nutritional or dietary constraints/monitoring
Orthodont	orthodontics
Orthotech	orthopedic technology
PhysApps	physical applications
PIR	postisometric relaxation
Psy	psychological-psychiatric adjuvant treatment
R	frequency of the injection treatment
Surg	surgical treatment
TENS	transcutaneous electrical nerve stimulation
ThE	therapeutic exercises
Urol	urological treatment
!	therapeutic ranking (+ to +++)

1 Introduction

■ Physiology of Pain Development

Worldwide, pain is the main reason for patients to seek medical care. It is much more difficult to encourage patients to enter treatment if a disorder is not accompanied by pain; hence, pain treatment is one of the main responsibilities of a therapist.

Regardless of whether the practitioner is a physician, physical therapist, naturopath, athletic coach, psychologist, or "green witch," the one who masters pain control the fastest and most effectively receives the most recognition.

In this respect, pain is not considered a homogenous formation but a collection of diverse sensations. Everybody knows light or stabbing pain, pain that can be precisely located, often involving the skin. This pain is transmitted via fast A delta fibers. On the other hand, there is the very dull, drawing pain, which is difficult to locate. This pain is transmitted via C fibers—unmyelinated, very slow acting nerve fibers. The first pain relay occurs in the spinal dorsal horn, where three different paths can be activated: the direct and shortest path to the spinal ventral horn, the path to the lateral horn, or the path via the medulla oblongata and brainstem ascending to the cortex can be chosen (**Fig. 1.1**).

Corresponding to the path chosen, very different reactions occur:

- The relay toward the ventral horn produces increased tension in the associated muscles. For example, this causes the hand to pull away when burning is sensed before pain is experienced.
- The relay toward the sympathetic complex in the lateral horn produces a vegetative response, that is, changes in blood circulation, connective tissue tension, or the pain threshold.
- The relay toward brainstem, thalamus, and cortex produces the actual pain sensation, including its individual interpretation, phenomena of pain projection, and highly complex facilitating and inhibiting concomitant phenomena.

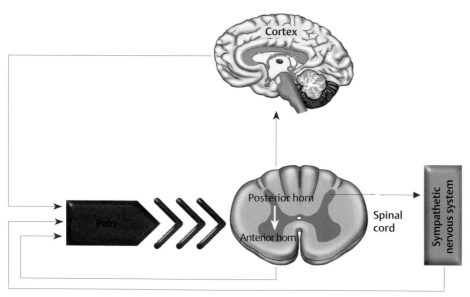

Fig. 1.1 Pain conduction and pain relay.

Therapeutic Possibilities

The therapeutic approaches for pain treatment are as multifarious as their therapists.

There are four fundamental possibilities:
- Pain treatment at the location of origin
- Pain treatment along the conduction pathways
- Pain treatment at the location of perception
- Pain treatment at the location of secondary effect

When a therapeutically effective stimulation is placed outside the location of pain origin and produces a reflexive reaction at the location of pain origin, one speaks of reflex therapy. Reflex therapies play a significant role in pain treatment. Examples for this type of therapy include manual medicine, acupuncture, physical-balneological treatments, and injection treatments.

There are frequent arguments about definitions—trigger points, reflex points, connective tissue zones, acupuncture points, spheres, and central pain are terms used for synonymous domains and distract from the fact that everyone refers to the same reflex phenomenon to achieve improvement.

Hereafter, we will not try to clarify this controversy, nor will we get lost in definition attempts ourselves, but would like to offer extracts from empirical knowledge about different areas that can be applied in daily practice.

Methods for Application of Local Anesthetics

In pain therapy through local anesthesia, four different application methods are distinguished:
1. Segmental therapy
2. Local therapy
3. Interference field therapy (special local therapy)
4. Blockage of conduction pathways

Segmental therapy is based on the fact that each neural segment of the spinal cord correlates developmentally with a particular zone of the skin and the connective tissue (dermatome), a particular zone of the musculature (myotome), and a particular zone of the skeletal system (sclerotome) (**Fig. 1.2**). Owing to the relay of neural fibers within the segment, interference can act crosswise. Thus, through treatment of the corresponding dermatome, for example, quaddle therapy, internal organs relating to the segment can be affected. Conversely, disorders of the correlating organs affect the respective myotomes and dermatomes. It is also possible to affect internal organs through the respective myotome or sclerotome.

Local therapy takes place directly at the site of the diseased tissue or organ. A typical example is the injection into tendons or muscle insertions, or injections in articular capsule dysfunctions (**Fig. 1.3**).

Interference field therapy treats zones with derailed tissue reaction. It is also a local therapy, generally treating injured and cicatricial areas, or areas affected by chronic inflammatory conditions. Unlike in the classic local therapy, these local interference fields (foci) can cause disorders away from the actual interference field without any neural connection. This type of chronic interference field can frequently be found in places of the tooth–mouth–pharynx space, for example, chronic tonsillitis or radicular foci. Surgical scars can also cause distant disturbances. Through injections under and around the focus, secondary disturbances can be eliminated (**Fig. 1.4**).

Local anesthesia to the conduction pathways includes injection and flooding of the neural path directly with a local anesthetic. In this case, pain conduction is interrupted through injection to the peripheral nerves (**Fig. 1.5**).

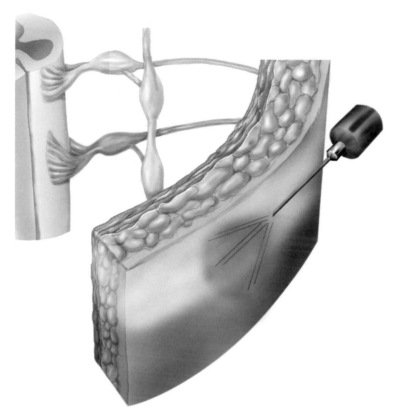

Fig. 1.2   Injection technique for segmental therapy. Note the segmental relationship of cutis, subcutis, and muscles with the corresponding spinal nerve.

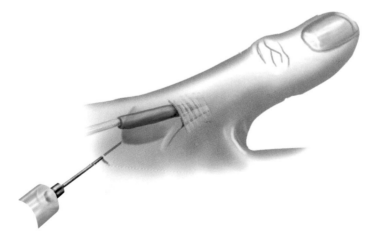

Fig. 1.3   Technique for local treatment.

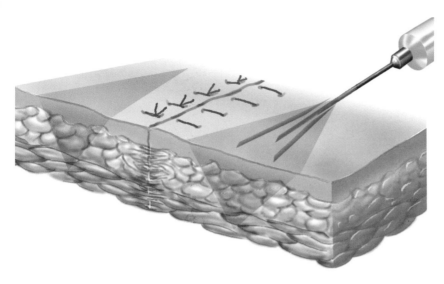

Fig. 1.4 Technique for treatment of an interference field by flooding of the localized interference field.

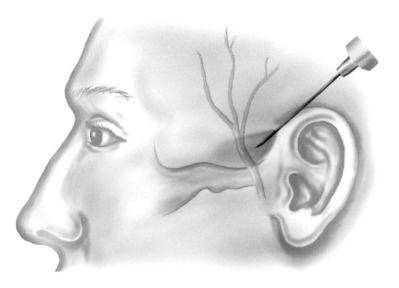

Fig. 1.5 Conduction pathway therapy; in this case, perineural flooding of a nerve. Arterial and venous pathways are treated in the same way. Caution: intra-neural and intra-arterial injections must be avoided.

■ Effects of Local Anesthetics

Even though our primary goal is pain elimination when injecting local anesthetics, we have to be aware that the local anesthetic produces several additional effects.

The most important effects of local anesthetics are listed as follows:

- Pain elimination
- Anti-inflammatory effect
- Sealing capillaries
- Antihistaminic effect
- Antiallergenic effect

■ Injection Techniques

Every therapist who begins the use of reflex therapy through the injection of local anesthetics will be quickly convinced of the efficacy of this method and include it in his or her repertoire of routine treatments. In spite of routine and everyday occurrence in regard to this treatment, each injection has to be performed with due diligence.

Injection therapy is one of the most effective reflex therapies. To perform injection therapy successfully, the following six principles have to be observed:

1. Legally, each injection is considered a grievous malicious injury, which is turned into "therapy" only through informing the patient and consent of the patient and lege artis performance of the therapist.
2. The most frequent and serious complications are infections; hence, cleaning and disinfection has to take place before every injection.
3. Skin cannot be sterilized! Skin cylinders are a focus of infection; therefore, the skin has to be tautened and the skin cylinder subcutaneously ejected.
4. The efficacy of the local anesthesia does not correspond to the amount of the local anesthetic used, but to the accuracy of the injection site.
5. Aspiration has to precede each injection to avoid intravascular administration.
6. Prevailing use of local anesthetics with amide structure (e.g., lidocaine) to reduce the risk of allergic reactions.

Obviously, disposable needles and disposable syringes must be used exclusively.

The needle should be as thin as possible and the syringe sufficiently long. Three different needle sizes (2 mL, 5 mL, and 10 mL) and seven different syringe sizes are suitable (**Table 1.1**).

Table 1.1 Cannulas

Color of cannula cone	Metric measuring units	Gauge and diameter
Gray	0.4 × 20 mm	72G, 0.25 in
Blue	0.6 × 30 mm	23G, 1.25 in
Black	0.7 × 30 mm	22G, 1.25 in
Green	0.8 × 50 mm	21G, 2 in
Yellow	0.9 × 40 mm	20G, 1.5 in
Yellow	0.9 × 70 mm	20G, 2.75 in
Yellow	0.9 × 90 mm	20G, 3.5 in

The local anesthetic is drawn into the syringe directly before the injection takes place. Storing syringes already filled with local anesthetic is not permitted due to the risk of infection. The cannula with which the local anesthetic is drawn from the vial is disposed of directly before the injection and is replaced with a new one. This decreases the risk of spreading pathogens. Also, the slightest contact with the vial damages the tip of modern cannulas. This causes a tear of the skin while the needle is being inserted, which results in additional pain.

The insertion site is sprayed with 70% alcohol or iodine substitute before the local anesthetic is drawn into the syringe. This extends the duration of exposure and increases the efficacy of the disinfection. In the case of intra-articular injections, an exposure time of at least 1 minute is required. The disinfectant is not wiped off, because pathogens would be wiped from the skin pores across the injection site.

Proper injection techniques help to avoid local side effects. We recommend a two-finger technique. After the injection site has been located, the surrounding area should be palpated (**Fig. 1.6a**). It

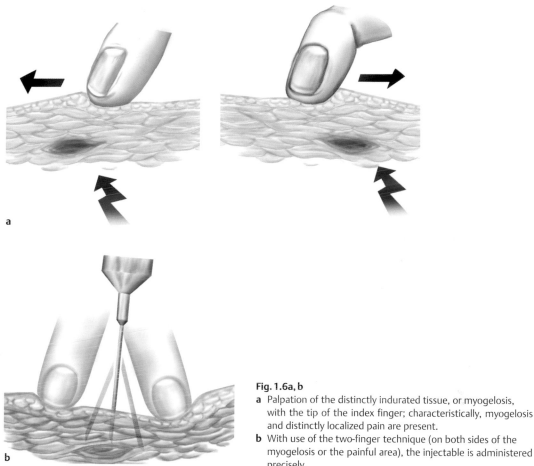

Fig. 1.6a, b
a Palpation of the distinctly indurated tissue, or myogelosis, with the tip of the index finger; characteristically, myogelosis and distinctly localized pain are present.
b With use of the two-finger technique (on both sides of the myogelosis or the painful area), the injectable is administered precisely.

must be ascertained that larger nerve or blood vessels do not cross the injection site. The skin is pretightened applying the two-finger technique (**Figs. 1.6b** and **1.7**). The needle must be thin and sufficiently long. Needle insertion is done quickly and only to the subcutaneous layer, where the skin cylinder is ejected. From there, the needle advances to the intended depth (**Fig. 1.8**). After the needle has been extracted, the site is first compressed with a swab and then sealed with a plaster. This way, the histoid repair mechanisms seal the injection channel rapidly.

Separate strict guidelines apply to intra-articular injections. High demands are placed on the space where the injection takes place. The spreading of pathogens should be avoided through proper scheduling and organization. Patients with secondary wound healing or similar sources of pathogens should not be treated in the same room.

The injection site is exposed to the disinfectant for at least 1 minute. The physician alone draws up the injectable into the syringe directly before the injection. This is done using a sterile technique, with the physician wearing gloves. Any type of conversation should be kept to a minimum during the injection process.

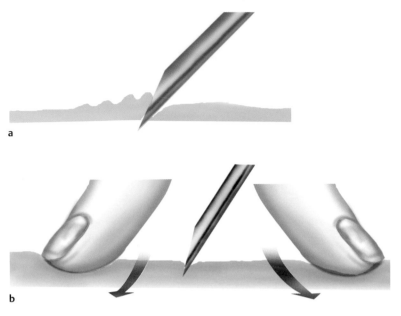

a

b

Fig. 1.7a, b
a Without pretightening of the skin, a "bulldozer effect" is created; the punched out skin cylinder covers a relatively large surface area.
b By pretightening the skin, the cannula pierces the skin without tiny skin folds being formed; the area of the punched-out skin cylinder is minimized.

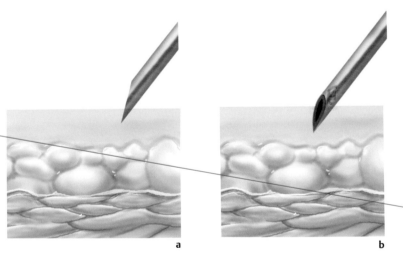

a

b

Fig. 1.8a–d
a Insertion into the pretightened skin.
b The cannula punches out the skin cylinder.

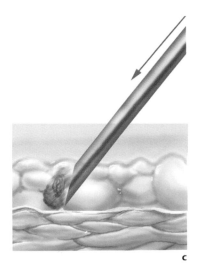
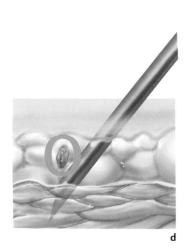

c

d

Fig. 1.8c,d
c Subcutaneous ejection of
   the skin cylinder.
d After ejection of the potential focus of infection, the
   needle is advanced subcutaneously.

Side Effects and Contraindications of Treatments with Local Anesthetics

The individual local anesthetics differ in their duration of effect, anesthetic potency, and also toxicity. In addition, they have differing allergic potential. Injection therapy requires repeated administration of local anesthetics, but an increasing number of the population is affected by allergic disorders. Therefore, we recommend the use of local anesthetics with amide structure (e.g., lidocaine). An overview of the duration of effect and toxicity is given in **Table 1.2**. Owing to the significantly increased risk, we principally do not recommend the addition of epinephrine.

We differentiate between local and systemic complications and side effects. Most local effects can be attributed to improper injection techniques.

The most frequent local side effects include:
• Vascular injury with secondary hemorrhage
• Local infection due to bacterial contamination
• Abacterial irritation caused by unsuitable additives
• Neural injury

Systemic side effects include:
• Toxic cardiovascular reactions (**Table 1.3**)
• Toxic central nervous system reactions
  (**Table 1.4**)
• Allergic reactions (**Table 1.5**)

Table 1.3   Cardiovascular toxicity

Symptoms	Therapy
Bradycardia	O_2 supply, intubation, artificial ventilation
Drop in blood pressure	Atropine and/or orciprenaline
Centralization	Arterenol
Asystole	Cardiopulmonary reanimation

Table 1.2   Duration of effect and relative toxicity of local anesthetics

Local anesthetic	Duration of effect	Maximum dose	Relative toxicity (1 for procaine)
Procaine	Up to 45 min	500 mg	1
Prilocaine	2–3 h	400 mg	4
Lidocaine	2–4 h	200 mg	4
Mepivacaine	2–4 h	300 mg	4
Bupivacaine	6–12 h	150 mg	10

Table 1.4   Central nervous system toxicity

Symptoms	Therapy
Numbness of tongue and mouth, metallic taste, tinnitus, vertigo, muscular twitches, slurred speech, deep, irregular breathing, vomiting	O_2 supply, diazepam (e.g., Valium), thiopental
Unconsciousness, cramps, apnea	Intubation, relaxation, regulation of metabolic acidosis (buffer agent $NaHCO_3$)

Dose:
Diazepam (e.g., Valium) 2.5–5 mg IV
Thiopental 25–50 mg IV, repeated injection, if applicable
Buffer agent ($NaHCO_3$) 150 meq, further adjustment after blood analysis

Table 1.5   Allergic reactions: symptoms, therapy, and dosage

Symptoms	Immediate measures	Dose
Flushing, urticaria	Peripheral venous access for high-flow-rate, O_2 supply, have emergency kit ready, alarm rescue chain	
Exanthema	In severe allergic incidents, immediate administration of epinephrine, as corticosteroids are effective only after 5–10 min	
Rhinitis	Epinephrine, 1 ampule 1 : 1000 = 1 mL = 1 mg	0.3 mg subcutaneously or 0.05–0.2 mg IV
Drop in blood pressure	Epinephrine/metered-dose inhaler (e.g., Adrenaline-Medihaler; 0.35 mg bitartrate per stroke)	Initially 1–2 strokes, repetition after 3–5 min
Tachycardia	H_1-receptor antagonists such as clemastine (e.g., Tavist, Tavegyl)	1–2 ampules (2–4 mg) IV
Arrhythmia	Dimetindene	1–2 ampules (4–8 mg) IV (= 0.1 mg/kg)
Vomiting	H_2-receptor antagonists such as cimetidine (e.g., Tagamet)	1–2 ampules (200–400 mg) IV
Bronchospasm	Corticosteroid dexamethasone	8–40 mg IV
Laryngeal edema	Prednisolone	250–1000 mg IV
Quincke edema	Volume therapy	Depending on the degree of severity, 2–3 L within the first 30 min is adequate; hydroxyethyl starch, full electrolyte solution

Indications for these reactions include:
• Restlessness, anxiety
• Drop in blood pressure, pulse deceleration
• Respiratory disorders, including laryngospasm

Local complications can generally be avoided by using the two-finger technique (see p.6 f).

Allergic and toxic reactions cannot always be avoided, even when proper techniques are applied. Local anesthetics must not be administered in the case of known hypersensitivity to them. Furthermore, contraindications must be considered.

General contraindications include:
• Blood coagulation disorders
• Allergic reactions to local anesthetics
• Severe cardiac conduction disturbance
• Infections at and near the injection site

When the first symptoms appear, proper response of the physician will prevent serious consequences

Table 1.6 Allergic reactions: severity, symptoms, and therapy

Degree of severity	Symptoms	Immediate measures
0	Localized cutaneous reaction	None
I	Skin reactions (flushing, urticaria, exanthema, rhinitis, conjunctivitis)	No additional LA injections, H_1/H_2-receptor antagonists
II	Drop in blood pressure, tachycardia, arrhythmia, nausea, vomiting, spasms of the digestive tract	No additional LA injections, corticosteroids, H_1/H_2-receptor antagonists, antidiuretic treatment, volume therapy
III	Shock, bronchospasm, laryngeal edema, Quincke edema	No additional LA injections, epinephrine subcutaneously, IV, metered-dose inhaler, corticosteroids, volume therapy
IV	Circulatory/respiratory arrest	No additional LA injections, cardiopulmonary resuscitation

LA, local anesthetic

(**Table 1.6**). After the patient has been positioned properly and oxygen supply has been provided (4 L/min), increasing restlessness is treated with sedatives (e.g., diazepam) and a venous access is put in place. In the case of light allergic reactions, administration of prednisolone sodium succinate (25–100 mg) is recommended, as well as clemastine (e.g., Tavist, Tavegyl) (2 mg) intravenously. Bradycardias are treated by cautious intravenous administration of atropine (0.5–1 mg). In the case of a slight drop in blood pressure, a saline infusion of etilefrine (e.g., Effortil) (one ampule) is recommended.

2 Head

■ Complex Pain

Temporal/Parietal Headache

Indications

- Temporal headache (yellow corresponds to the area of radiation)
- Parietal headache (yellow and blue corresponds to the area of radiation)

Differential Diagnoses

- Temporal (yellow pain area)
  Disorders of the mandibular joints and ears, as well as pain referred from the base of the lung, heart, and pericardium
- Parietal (yellow and blue pain area)
  Headache due to hypertension and hypotension as well as pain referred from disorders of the pylorus and the intestines

Material

- Local anesthetic: 2–3 mL
- Needle: 0.4 × 20 mm

Technique

- The temporal artery is palpated and shielded with the palpating finger. The needle is inserted in front of and behind the artery into the temporalis muscle.
- Supraorbitally, the notch at the center of the bone above the eye is palpated and the needle is inserted cranially at an angle until bone contact is made.

Risks

- Injury to the temporal artery, if the artery is not shielded with the palpating finger, and to the supraorbital artery (avoid by attempting aspiration prior to injection).
- If there is a galvanic response across the anterolateral part of the skull when the anesthetic is being injected into the anterior temporal region, the needle is inserted slightly more ventrally to avoid injury to the temporoparietal nerve.

Concomitant Therapies

- Manual mobilization of the temporomandibular joint, if indicated
- Complemented by temporalis relaxation and relaxation therapy

Remarks

Ask patients about grinding teeth at night, blockage, and/or galvanic pain when chewing (if applicable, orthodontic bite guard).

! +++
R 2–3 times a week
MM, PIR, Orthodont

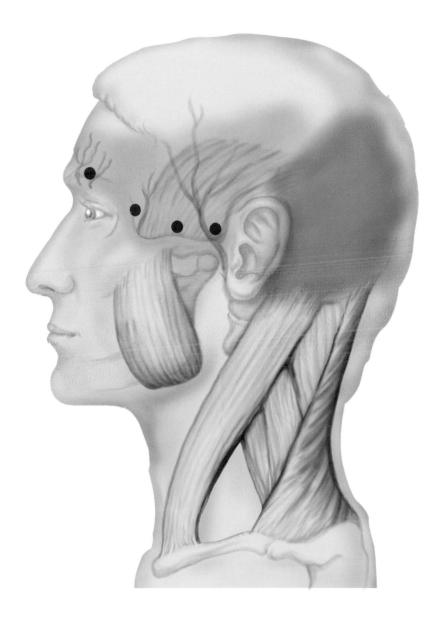

● Primarily indicated injection points

● Complementary point

▢ Area of pain distribution

Occipitoparietal Headache

Indications

- Occipitoparietal headache (blue corresponds to the pain area)

Differential Diagnoses

- Craniovertebral joints, disorders in the area of the cervical vertebrae, disorders of the nasal and maxillary sinuses and the pharyngeal tonsils
- Referred pain from liver, intestines, ovaries, and testicles

Material

- Local anesthetic: 3 mL
- Needle: 0.4 × 20 mm

Technique

- The insertion of the sternocleidomastoid and the palpable protuberance of the mastoid process is located; less than 1 finger width behind the posterior base of the ear the needle is inserted vertically until bone contact is made; the second injection is performed 2 finger widths toward the occiput where the muscles of the neck insert (directly above the hairline).
- Complementary injection sites are located at and between the caudal insertions of the sternocleidomastoid at the end of the clavicle and the superior edge of the sternum.

Risks

- The occipital insertion point away from the ear is close to the course of the occipital vein and artery. Avoid intra-arterial injection through prior aspiration.
- For the injection at the distal insertion of the sternocleidomastoid, the needle is inserted almost 1 cm. To recognize injury to the jugular or transverse cervical vein in time and to prevent excessively deep injection, aspiration is mandatory.

Concomitant Therapies

- Complemented by traction treatments, for example, Glisson traction and manual mobilization techniques
- Acupressure
- Transcutaneous electrical nerve stimulation therapy
- Chiropractic treatment

Remarks

- Severe occipitoparietal headache in the morning indicates faulty sleeping position.
- Abdominal sleeping position must be avoided. Try special neck cushions, if applicable.

!++
R 2 times a week, up to 3 weeks
ThE, MM, Acu, TENS, Chiro, Orthotech

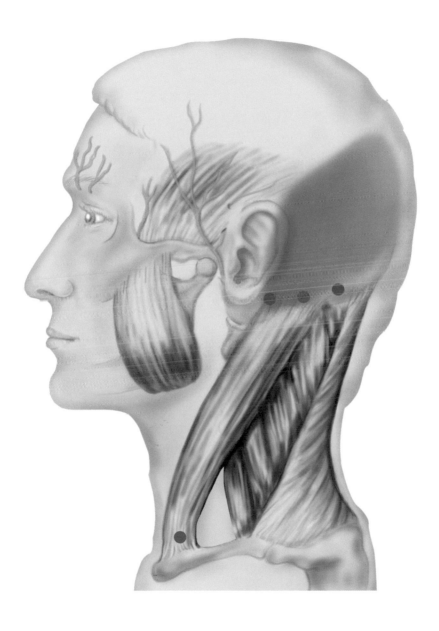

● Primarily indicated injection points

● Complementary point

Parietal Lock

Indications

- Chronic parietal headache
- Pulsating temporal headache
- Pain accompanying ear disorders
- Tension headache
- Headache triggered by hormones
- Posttraumatic headache

Differential Diagnoses

- Disorders of the mandibular joints, upper and lower jaw, nasal and frontal sinuses, disorders involving the zygomatic arch, inflammatory changes of the scalp

Material

- Local anesthetic: 4–5 mL
- Needle: 0.4 × 20 mm

Technique

- It is recommended that the parietal lock be implemented from two separate injection sites. The first injection site is located by placing the palpating finger slightly less than 1 cm supraorbital and carefully moving it toward the upper rim of the ear, where it will slide into a shallow depression. At this site, the needle is inserted toward the anterior upper rim of the ear. At the same time, the other hand tightens the skin toward the forehead. Now the needle is advanced parallel to the skull, almost up to the anterior rim of the ear. The local anesthetic is injected at intervals while the needle is being retracted.
- The second injection takes place approximately 3 cm behind the posterior base of the ear. At the upper edge of the lateral occiput, the needle is inserted toward the ear. From there it is advanced until it almost reaches the posterior base of the ear. The local anesthetic is injected at intervals while the needle is being retracted.

Risks

- The frontal arch of the superficial temporal artery may be injured in the area of the anterior injection site. Fortunately, the pulsation of the artery is easily palpable. Aspiration prior to injection avoids unintentional intravascular administration.
- Injury to the auricle must be avoided during injection behind the ear.

Concomitant Therapies

- In ear disorders, a quaddle may be placed at the Ear Gate, acupuncture point TB-21.
- In migraines, an additional injection may be performed at the exit of the supraorbital nerve.
- In tension headaches, autogenic training, biofeedback therapy, muscle relaxation techniques, for example, according to Jacobson, acupressure, and reflexotherapy of the feet are recommended.
- If applicable, systemic myotonolysis by means of medication.

! ++(+)
R 2 times a week, up to 4 weeks
Acu, Med, Auto, BFB, MR

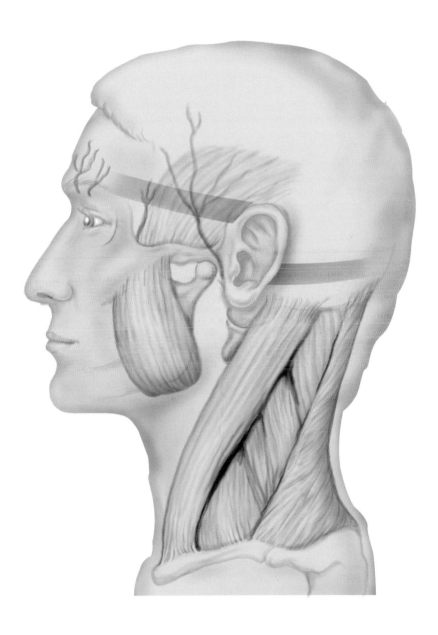

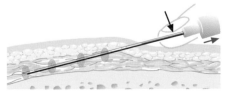

Occipital Headache

Indications

- Occipital headache, tension headache, headache involving the area of the forehead and eyes, occipitosacral pain patterns
- Distal therapy for pancreatic disorders

Material

- Local anesthetic: unilateral 3 mL, bilateral 6 mL
- Needle: 0.4 × 20 mm

Technique

- With the head in the neutral position, injection takes place 3 cm superior and 3 cm lateral to the first palpable spinous process. This area is usually sensitive to pressure. The needle is inserted vertically and advanced until bone contact is made.
- The second injection takes place 1.5 cm laterally and caudally of first injection to a depth of 1.5–2 cm, where the local anesthetic is administered medially and laterally in a fan-shaped pattern.
- The third injection takes place slightly next to the median line, superior to the first palpable spinous process, to a depth of 1.5–2 cm. The final injection takes place subcutaneously 3 cm posterior to the superior base of the ear. The needle is inserted 3–4 mm only.

Risks

- Use of excessively long cannulas may lead to insertion into the vertebral canal and injection into the cistern magna.
- Injection into the atlantooccipital membrane with severely painful sequelae. In this case, very strong resistance can be felt during the injection and the needle should be withdrawn a few millimeters.
- The patient should be informed that anesthesia of the greater occipital nerve causes a sensation of numbness in the area of the posterior scalp.
- Unintentional injections into the occipital artery are avoided through prior aspiration.

Concomitant Therapies

- Postisometric relaxation treatments to the neck extensors
- Extension of the cervical spine through manual therapy or Glisson traction
- In headaches that occur predominantly in the morning, prescription of neck cushions
- Suboccipital application of transcutaneous electrical nerve stimulation
- Relaxation techniques
- Biofeedback therapy
- If applicable, physical therapy, chiropractic treatment

! +++
R 2–3 times a week, up to 3 months
PIR, MM, PhysApps, BFB, Psy, Chiro

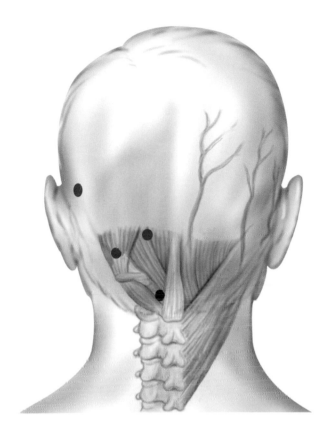

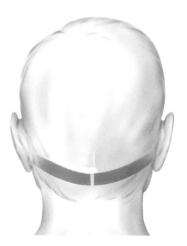

● Primarily indicated injection points

Area of pain distribution

Pain in the Region of the Ear

Indications

- Adjuvant treatment in the case of otogenic verti-go and tinnitus, radiating pain from chronically recurring otitis, and disorders referring from other areas, particularly the sternocleidomas-toid

Differential Diagnoses

- Disorders of the mandibular joint and bite anomalies
- Vertebrogenic pain projecting from segment C 3 or C 7

Material

- Local anesthetic: 2–3 mL
- Needle: 0.4 × 20 mm

Technique

- The injection sites behind the ear are located directly superior to the mastoid process. The injection sites in front of the ear are located 1.5–2 finger widths superior to the posterior sites, on an imaginary line between the eyebrow and the tragus. The needle is inserted vertically and advanced until bone contact is made. The needle is then retracted 1–2 mm and 0.5 mL of a local anesthetic is injected.
- In front of the ear, at the level of the tragus, a small depression can be found that corresponds to acupuncture point SI-19. Here, the needle is inserted vertically 0.5 mm and 0.5 mL of a local anesthetic is injected.
- From the superior border of the auricle toward the orbital cavity, three points are located 1 cm apart. They compose the path of the masseter. The needle is inserted vertically 1 cm and 0.5 mL of a local anesthetic is injected.

Risks

- At the injection site corresponding to acupuncture point SI-19, in front of the tragus, the facial nerve may be anesthetized if the needle is advanced excessively.
- If the temporal artery is injured during injection, large hematomas may form in the temporalis area; therefore, aspiration prior to injection is mandatory.

Concomitant Therapies

- Especially in edematous tissue changes around the ear, treatment with cantharis plaster is rec-ommended.
- In chronic otitis, injection therapy is only an adjuvant treatment and cannot replace the treatment of the inflammatory condition of the inner ear.
- In tinnitus, adjuvant cryogenic friction massage at the insertion site of the sternocleidomastoid and chiropractic treatment has proven success-ful.
- In chronic inflammatory ear disorders, adjuvant enzymatic treatments, including lysozyme and bromelain, are utilized.

! ++
R 2 times a week, up to 3 weeks
Med, FMA, Chiro

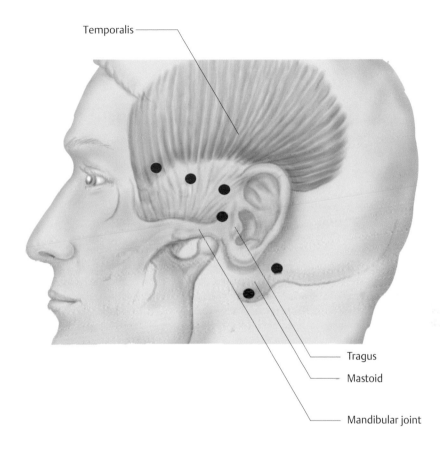

Temporalis

Tragus

Mastoid

Mandibular joint

● Primarily indicated injection points

Area of pain distribution

■ Treatment through Muscles, Tendons, and Ligaments

Temporalis

Indications

- Parietal pain and pain radiating toward the ear
- Chronic pain in the region of the upper teeth, including hyperpathia of the teeth

Differential Diagnoses

- Retrobulbar processes
- Intracranial disorders
- Vasomotor and tension headaches
- Dysfunctions of the masticatory system

Material

- Local anesthetic: 3 mL
- Needle: 0.4 × 20 mm

Technique

- The injection sites are located on an imaginary line between the superior border of the auricle and the eyebrow. The needle is inserted vertically 0.5–1 cm. A local anesthetic (0.5–1 mL) is injected at each site.
- Alternatively, the needle is inserted tangentially from the superior border of the lateral eyebrow toward the superior border of the auricle. While the needle is being retracted, the local anesthetic is injected at intervals (see parietal lock injection, p. 16).

Risks

- Injury to the temporal vein and artery
- Anesthesia of the temporal nerve, including superficial anesthesia of the parietal region extending toward the eye

Concomitant Therapies

- Acupressure is recommended, especially in the case of hypertonic affections of the temporalis.
- With use of appropriate equipment, biofeedback therapy is also highly effective.

! ++
R 1–2 times a week, up to 6 weeks
Acu, BFB

Temporalis

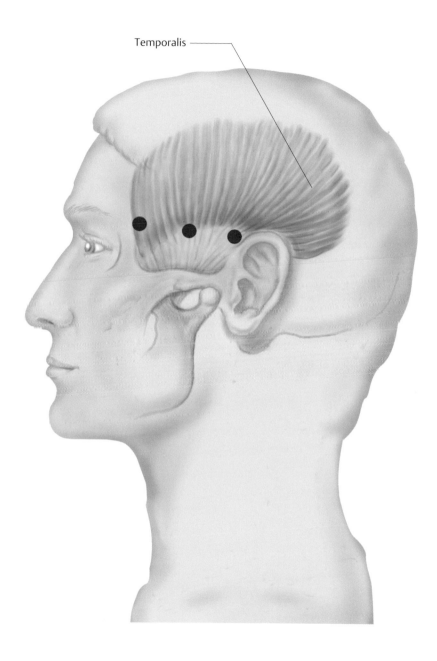

● Primarily indicated injection points

　 Area of pain distribution

Masseter and Mandibular Joint

Indications

- Particularly, pain originating in the masseter and radiating into the lower jaw and the mandibular angle. Hypersensitive reactions result in the area of the lower teeth as well as in the area of the canines of the upper jaw.
- Occasionally, pain radiates into the center of the face toward the nose.
- Affections of the mandibular joint are characterized by pain during mastication, accompanied by pressure sensitivity above the joint.

Material

- Local anesthetic: 1–2 mL for the masseter, 1 mL for the mandibular joint
- Needle: 0.4 × 20 mm

Technique

- The mandibular joint can be palpated in front of the ear at the level of the tragus. While the patient opens and closes the mouth, the joint can be palpated precisely. The needle is inserted vertically 0.5–1 cm.
- The two insertion sites located near the mandibular joint are found at the level of the masseter muscle belly while the patient clenches his or her teeth. The depth of insertion is 1 cm. At each site, 0.5 mL of a local anesthetic is injected.
- The two injection sites along the zygomatic arch are located near the zygomatic bone. The site closer to the ear is located at the lower edge of the zygomatic arch, barely 3 finger widths in front of the tragus. The site closer to the nose is located by palpating along the zygomatic arch. At the end of the arch, the finger dips into a slight depression, which indicates the insertion site. The needle is inserted vertically 0.5 cm.

Risks

- The maxillary artery can be injured through injections in the area of the mandibular joint and injections into the masseter at the lower edge of the zygomatic arch if the needle is advanced excessively. The course of the maxillary artery varies considerably and aspiration prior to injection is vital.

Concomitant Therapies

- Postisometric relaxation treatments of the masseter as well as mobilization treatment of the mandibular joint, in particular, manual therapy above the mandible.
- In bite anomalies, orthodontic co-treatment.
- If the patient continuously grinds his or her teeth at night, a bite guard may be indicated at night to relieve tension in the masseter.

> ! +++
> R 2 times a week, up to 4 weeks
> PIR, Orthotech, MM

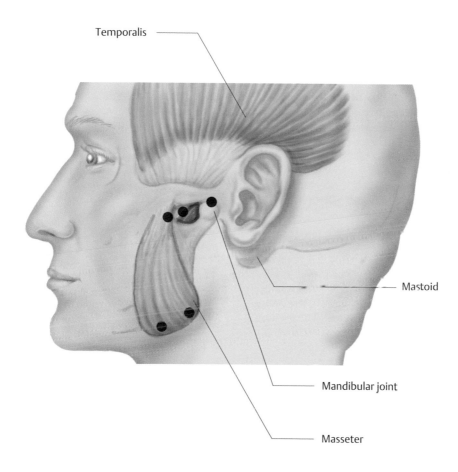

Temporalis

Mastoid

Mandibular joint

Masseter

● Primarily indicated injection points

  Area of pain distribution

■ Treatment through Nerves

Supraorbital Nerve

Indications

• Chronic affections of the frontal sinuses and unilateral frontal headache

Differential Diagnoses

• Glaucoma
• Retrobulbar affections. Caution: tumors

Material

• Local anesthetic: 0.5 mL
• Needle: 0.4 × 20 mm

Technique

• At the center of the orbital cavity, the superior
edge of the orbit is palpated with the finger
moving toward the nose. The palpable supraorbital notch indicates the insertion site. The
needle is inserted cranially at a 45° angle and
advanced until bone contact is made. After the
needle has been retracted approximately 1–2 mm,
0.5 mL of a local anesthetic is injected.

Risks

• Intra-arterial injection into the supraorbital
artery; therefore, aspiration is vital prior to the
injection.

Concomitant Therapies

• Additional injections or acupuncture along the
bladder channel, especially BL-2 and BL-8, as
well as acupuncture to the stomach channel
(ST-8)
• Large-area application of peppermint oil on the
forehead and temples achieves good results.

! ++
R once a week, up to 8 weeks
Acu, Med

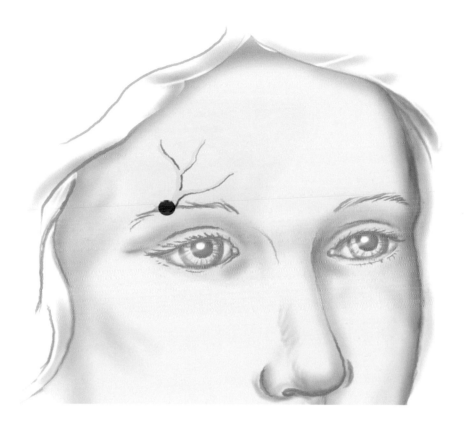

● Primarily indicated injection points

░ Area of pain distribution

Infraorbital Nerve

Indications

- Pain in the central region of the face near the second (maxillary) branch of the trigeminal nerve, as well as chronic affections of the paranasal and maxillary sinuses

Differential Diagnoses

- Chronic suppurative inflammation in the maxillary region, which requires dental examination

Material

- Local anesthetic: 0.5 mL
- Needle: 0.4 × 20 mm

Technique

- In this condition, several techniques can be applied, some transorally others transcutaneously. The insertion near the point where the nerve exits the bone has proven to be one of the simplest and therapeutically most effective techniques.
- The palpating finger locates the center of the inferior edge of the orbit. From there, the insertion site is located 1 cm caudally and 1 cm medially. The needle is inserted at an angle in the direction of the nose and advanced 1–1.5 cm.

Risks

- Intra-arterial injection into the infraorbital artery; therefore, aspiration is vital prior to injection.
- The risk of an intravenous injection into the facial vein must also be avoided through prior aspiration.

Concomitant Therapies

- Concomitant treatment by an otolaryngologist, if applicable
- Anti-inflammatory inhalation therapy in the case of irritation of the paranasal sinuses
- Cryomassage

! ++
R once a week, up to 8 weeks
ENT, MA, Med

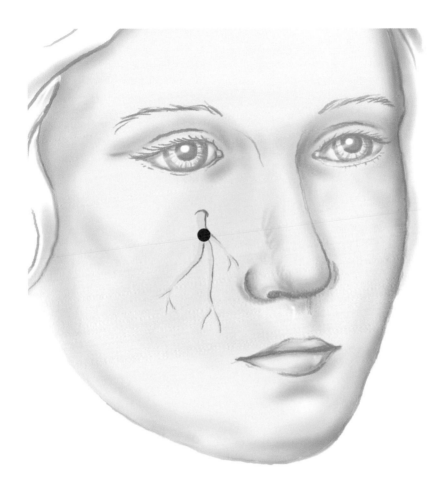

● Primarily indicated injection points

Area of pain distribution

■ Treatment through the Skin

"Crown of Thorns"

Indications

- Chronic headache of unknown origin, as well as tension headache
- Adjuvant treatment in the case of vegetative dysfunctions, cerebral circulatory disorders, and pain following concussion

Material

- Local anesthetic: 3 mL
- Needle: 0.4 × 20 mm

Technique

- Along the line of the greatest head circumference, injections are performed every 3 cm; 0.5 mL of a local anesthetic is injected each time. Part of the injectable is placed as a quaddle and the rest is injected into the scalp after the needle has been advanced a further 2–3 mm.

Risks

- None

Concomitant Therapies

- Depending on the indication regarding tension headaches, special relaxation techniques apply, for example, progressive relaxation technique according to Jacobson and biofeedback therapy.
- Transcutaneous application of essential peppermint oil along the forehead and on the parietal area

! ++
R 2–3 times a week, up to 6 weeks
MR, BFB, Med

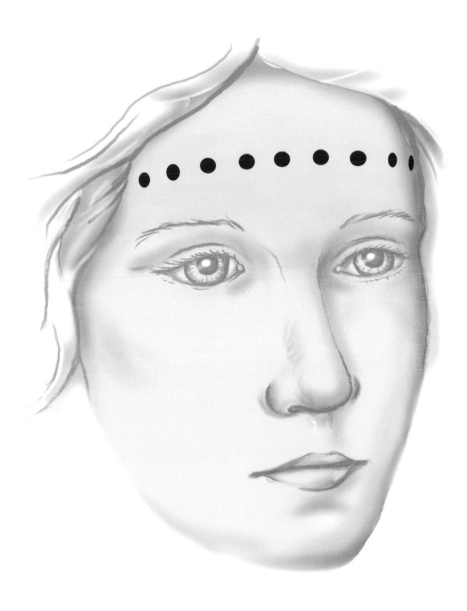

● Primarily indicated injection points

Area of pain distribution

3 Cervical Spine

■ Complex Pain

Nonspecific Neck Pain

Indications

- Pain in the area of the posterior cervical spine without point of maximal intensity, not related to specific muscles, frequently including hyperpathia of the skin
- Pain when actively flexing the neck, increasing against resistance
- Increased pain with passive flexion

Differential Diagnoses

- Arthrosis of the cervical facet joints
- Myalgia of the deep neck extensors
- Interspinous neoarthrosis (pain is absent during passive flexion)

Material

- Local anesthetic: 10 mL
- Needle: 0.4 × 20 mm

Technique

- The tips of the spinous processes are marked. The injections sites are located 2 cm paramedially to the right and to the left, at the level of the tips of the spinous processes. The needle is inserted vertically.
- The depth of insertion is 1–2 cm and each injection site receives 0.5 mL of a local anesthetic.

Risks

- None

Concomitant Therapies

- Stretching of the posterior cervical muscles
- Glisson traction
- Local heat application
- Neck compress
- Progressive muscle relaxation

! +++
R 1–2 times a week
MM, Auto, BFB, Chiro, TENS

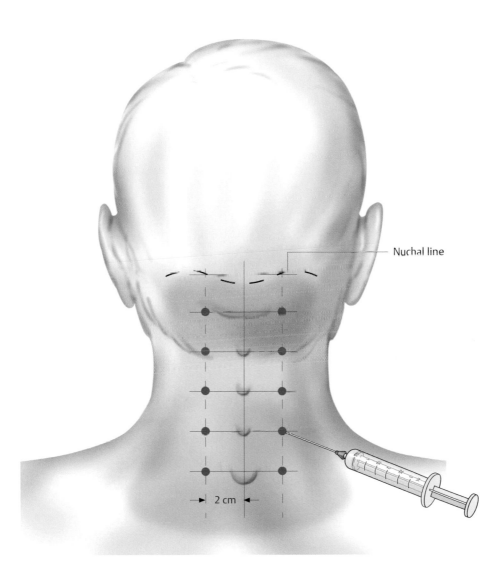

Nuchal line

2 cm

Interspinous Neoarthrosis / Irritation of the Interspinales

Indications

- Distinct segmental pain in the posterior neck, increasing during active and passive neck flexion and remaining unchanged during neck extension

Differential Diagnoses

- Tendinosis at the insertion of the deep neck muscles
- Irritation of the vertebral joints

Material

- Local anesthetic: 2 mL
- Needle: 0.4 × 20 mm

Technique

- The patient is seated, shoulders are relaxed, and the cervical spine is extended. The spinous process of C7 is palpated; from there palpation moves upward until the painful segment is identified. To confirm the finding, the neck is passively extended, which must produce the characteristic pain.
- The injection site is located between the palpable tips of the spinous processes. The needle is inserted at a 20° angle cranially. The depth of insertion is 1.5–2 cm. Distinct resistance is felt when the nuchal ligament is penetrated.

Risks

- Injections into the nuchal ligament frequently produce intense pain; therefore, injection is discontinued in cases of high resistance.
- Advancing the needle excessively creates the risk of an epidural injection. The extended position of the neck allows the interlaminar gap to widen. Therefore, longer needles must not be used.

Concomitant Therapies

- Passive traction of the cervical spine
- Orthopedic brace extending the cervical spine
- Administration of NSAIDs with systemic effect

! ++
R once a week
MM, Orthotech, Med, Auto

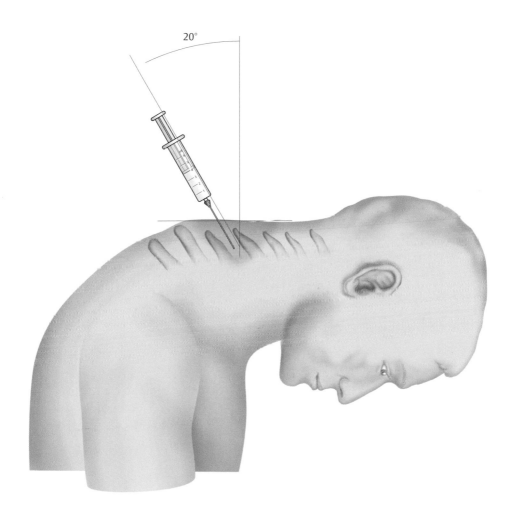

■ Treatment through Muscles, Tendons, and Ligaments

Levator Scapulae

Indications

- Pain in the posterior shoulder, frequently non-specific and dull, cannot be exactly localized by the patient
- Characteristic trigger point in the area of the muscle's superior border at the tip of the medial scapula, frequently radiating across the superior border of the trapezius

Differential Diagnoses

- Facet irritation in the C5/C6 segment
- Irritation of the suprascapular nerve with compression in the area of the suprascapular notch caused by the transverse scapular ligament
- Costovertebral joint block at the level of T3

Material

- Local anesthetic: 3 mL
- Needle: 0.4 × 20 mm

Technique

- The tip of the medial scapula is located and is usually very sensitive to pressure. The most important injection site is in the center of this painful area. Two additional injection sites are located on a transverse line in the craniomedial direction, each 3 cm apart.
- Each site receives 1 mL of a local anesthetic injected 2 cm deep.

Risks

- None

Concomitant Therapies

- Cryogenic friction massage at the insertion site of the levator scapulae
- Local treatment, for example, along the course of the levator scapulae, with moist heat
- Manual therapy, applying gliding mobilization of the scapulothoracic gliding plane
- Behavioral therapy (frequent cause: mental stress syndromes and anxieties, patients pull their shoulders up to their ears)
- Medical exercise therapy

! +++
R 2 times a week, up to 6 weeks
MM, PhysApps, Psy, MET

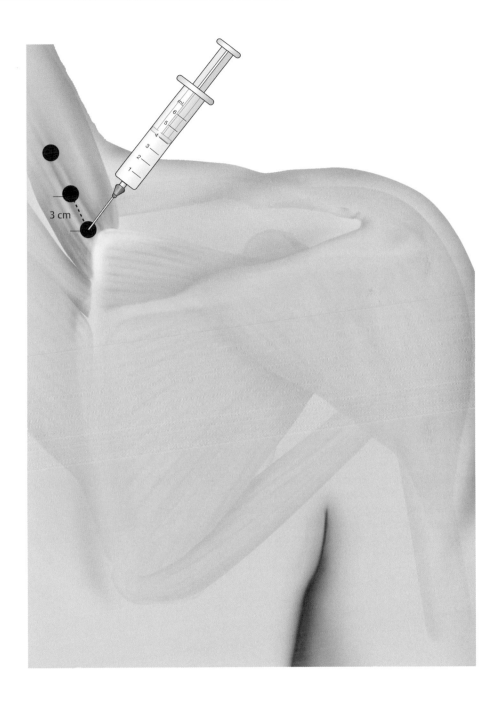

3 cm

● Primarily indicated injection points

▪ Area of pain distribution

Sternocleidomastoid

Indications

- Motion-dependent headache on the lateral aspect of the head, frequently located in the area of the mastoid process and the ear, radiating
- Simultaneous supraorbital and frontal pain

Possible Concomitant Symptoms

- Bilateral watery eyes
- Vertigo
- Pain increases when the head is bent to the opposite side and rotated to the same side

Differential Diagnoses

- Vascular headache
- Trigeminal neuralgia

Material

- Local anesthetic: 4 mL
- Needle: 0.4 × 20 mm

Technique

- The sternocleidomastoid is located and is taken between the thumb and the index finger. The muscle is divided into five equal segments between the origin and the insertion. The insertion sites are located in the center of each segment. The needle is inserted vertically and advanced 1.5 cm. Each injection site receives 1 mL of a local anesthetic.
- For the injection into the cervical head, the sternocleidomastoid is marked halfway between the insertion and the origin. Here, the needle is inserted vertically at the posterior border of the muscle and advanced 3 cm. At this depth, 2 mL of a local anesthetic is administered.

Risks

- The jugular vein can be punctured if the needle is inserted too deep.
- Therefore, aspiration is mandatory before injection.

Concomitant Therapies

- Postisometric relaxation
- Cryotherapy with passive stretches of the sternocleidomastoid
- Orthopedic brace to support the cervical spine

! +
R once a week
PIR, PhysApps, MET

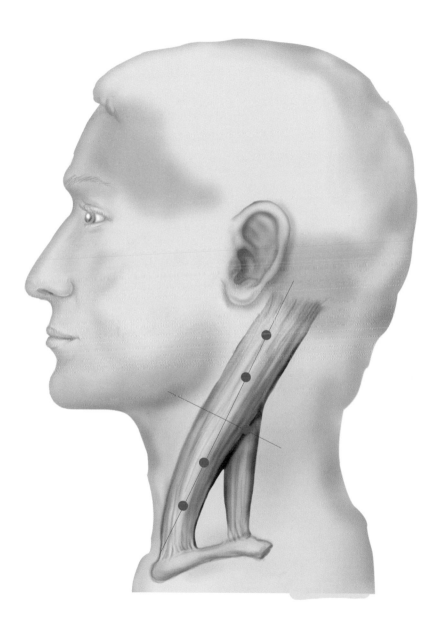

Trapezius

Indications

- Nonspecific shoulder–neck–arm pain extending along the top of the shoulder
- Adjuvant treatment in the case of tension headache and degenerative cervical syndrome
- Adjuvant treatment in the case of obstructive respiratory disorders

Differential Diagnoses

- Radicular symptoms
- Nerve compartment syndromes

Material

- Local anesthetic: 5 mL
- Needle: 0.4 × 20 mm

Technique

- Along a line that runs 3–4 cm parallel to the top of the shoulder, a local anesthetic is injected vertically every 3 cm.
- A local anesthetic (0.2–0.5 mL) is injected intracutaneously.
- After the needle has been advanced 1 cm, 0.5 mL of a local anesthetic is injected.

Risks

- In the central injection area, excessively deep needle insertion into the pleural dome can cause a pneumothorax; therefore, the recommended depth of insertion cannot be exceeded.

Concomitant Therapies

- Local heat application
- Medical exercise therapy, relaxing massages
- Electrotherapy treatments that lower the muscle tone

! ++
R 3 times a week, up to 8 weeks
PhysApps, ThE, MET, Med

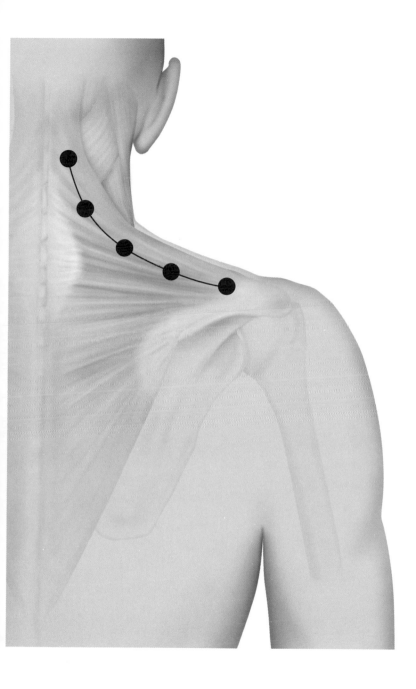

● Primarily indicated injection points

Area of pain distribution

Rectus Capitis Posterior Major and Minor

Indications

- Unilateral or bilateral occipital pain, increasing when the head is bent backward against resistance and during passive flexion of the superior aspect of the neck
- Distinct pressure sensitivity approximately 2 cm inferior to the nuchal line

Differential Diagnoses

- Occipital neuralgia differs in pain location. Pain originating in the rectus capitis posterior radiates along the occiput to the ear. Pain originating in the occipital nerve radiates across the occiput and skull all the way to the frontal orbital region.

Material

- Local anesthetic: 6 mL
- Needle: 0.6 × 30 mm

Technique

- On a horizontal line 2 cm inferior to the nuchal line, the injection sites are located 1, 2, and 3 cm lateral to the median line.
- The needle is inserted vertically and advanced 1.5 cm. Each injection site receives 1 mL of a local anesthetic.

Risks

- Anesthesia of parts of the lesser and the greater occipital nerve.
- The patient must be informed that in the area supplied by the occipital nerve, a sensation of numbness may occur.

Concomitant Therapies

- Trigger points in the area are usually activated by tipping the head back above the cervical spine. Therefore, visual impairments, such as unsuitable spectacle frames or not wearing prescription spectacles in cases of near-sightedness, are frequent causes of this pain. Bad posture at the workplace is another cause.
- Topical heat application
- Acupuncture
- Infiltration and passive neck extension

Note Orthopedic neck braces are perceived to be more annoying than helpful because the superior border exerts direct pressure onto all cervical muscles.

! ++
R 1–2 times a week
MM, TENS, Med, Orthotech, Acu, PhysApps

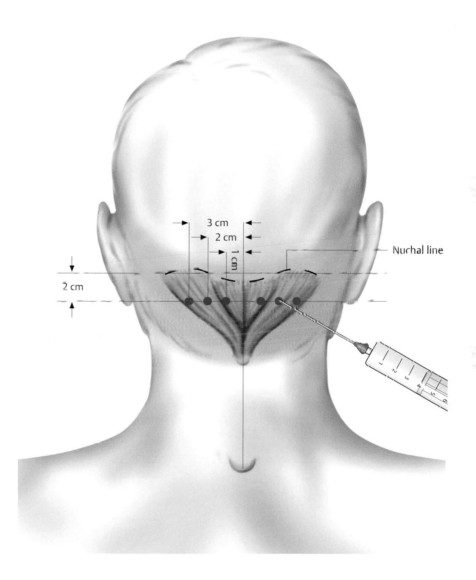

■ Treatment through Nerves

Greater and Lesser Occipital Nerve

Indications

- Neuralgias and irritations of the greater and the lesser occipital nerve
- Characteristic occipital headache radiating across the scalp to the supraorbital region
- Distinct irritation at the exit site of the greater occipital nerve during local palpation
- Headache remains unchanged during passive flexion and extension of the neck

Differential Diagnoses

- Irritation of the rectus capitis posterior major and minor (increasing during active flexion of the neck)

Material

- Local anesthetic: 3 mL on each side
- Needle: 0.6 × 30 mm

Technique

- The patient is in a prone or seated position. The nuchal line is palpated. A vertical auxiliary line is drawn, 1 cm inferiorly. Four centimeters lateral to the median line, the needle is inserted horizontally, parallel to the nuchal line. One centimeter into the tissue, several injections of 0.5 mL of a local anesthetic are administered, 1–2 cm apart. This creates an infiltration band parallel to the nuchal line.
- The patient is informed that anesthesia of the occipital nerve causes temporary numbness in the posterior skull.

Risks

- None

Concomitant Therapies

- Relaxation therapies (e.g., autogenic training)
- Administration of analgesics with systemic effect
- Morning headaches are frequently caused by false sleeping position of the head, such as an excessively hard or voluminous pillow.

! +++
R 1–2 times a week
Auto, BFB, TENS, Acu, Med

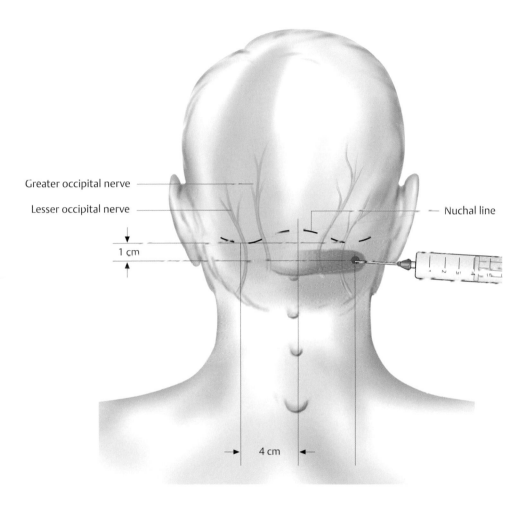

Greater occipital nerve

Lesser occipital nerve

Nuchal line

1 cm

4 cm

■ Treatment through Joints

Cervical Vertebral Joints of the C4–C6 Segments

Indications

- Arthrosis of the vertebral joints causing inflammation or irritation of the vertebral joints

Differential Diagnoses

- Interspinous neoarthrosis
- Myogelosis in the deep neck muscles
- Cervical radiculitis

Material

- Local anesthetic: 2 mL for each facet and side
- Needle: 0.8 × 50 mm

Technique

- The patient is seated with the neck slightly extended by 10° (if the neck is extended further, the interlaminar gap widens, which creates the risk of a peridural injection).
- The median line and the spinous processes are marked. An additional auxiliary line is drawn 2 cm paramedially.
- The injection sites are located on the paramedian auxiliary line between the palpable tips of the spinous processes. The needle is inserted vertically and advanced until bone contact is made. Aspiration takes place prior to injection of 2 mL of a local anesthetic per facet.
- Intra-articular placement of the needle is often not precise. Pericapsular injection suffices to achieve the desired therapeutic result.

Risks

- Peridural injection; therefore, the neck must be inclined slightly to avoid widening the interlaminar gap.
- Injection into the deep cervical and the vertebral artery. It is vital to repeat aspiration while the needle is being advanced.

Anesthesia of the Spinal Nerve

- If the needle is inserted too far laterally or advanced in a transverse-lateral direction, the spinal nerve can be anesthetized. It is necessary to ensure that the needle makes bone contact prior to injection of the local anesthetic.

Note After making bone contact and injecting the local anesthetic, the needle needs to be replaced before injecting the local anesthetic into the next vertebral joint because the tip of the needle is now dull owing to the contact with the bone.

! ++
R once a week
Orthotech, PhysApps, MM, TENS, Med

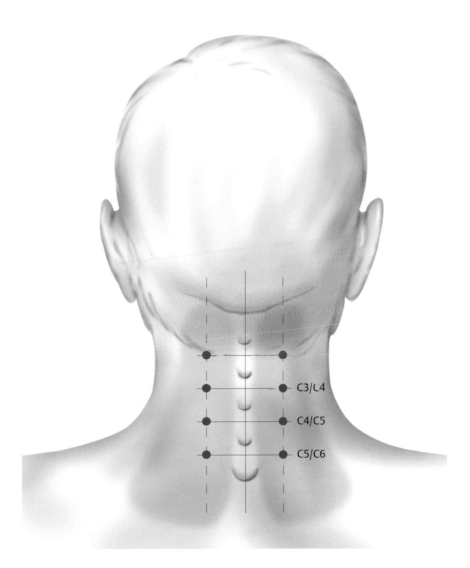

4 Upper Extremities

▪ Complex Pain

Anterior Shoulder and Subacromial Pain

Indications

- Shoulder–arm pain
- Humeroscapular periarthritis
- Degenerative changes in the rotator cuff
- Omarthrosis
- Musculotendinous overload
- Frozen shoulder
- Referred pain symptoms arising from cardiac disorders

Material

- Local anesthetic: 5–7 mL
- Needle: 0.6 × 60 mm

Technique

- The acromioclavicular joint is located through palpation while the arm is placed in slight internal rotation. From there, the insertion site is barely 1.5 cm inferolaterally. The tip of the needle points transversely from anterolateral in the posteromedial direction. The needle is advanced 2.5–3 cm until bone contact is made. The local anesthetic is administered successively while the needle is being retracted.
- Now, 3–4 cm medially at the same level, the usually painful coracoid process is located. The needle is advanced until bone contact is made. Then, the needle is slightly retracted and advanced again inferiorly for 1 cm. Following aspiration, the local anesthetic is injected.
- The injection slightly inferolateral to the acromioclavicular joint completes the therapeutic triangle. The needle first makes bone contact, is slightly retracted, and 0.5 mL of a local anesthetic is injected.
- Additionally, the insertion of the ligament at the superior edge of the coracoid process can be flooded with the injectable. If pain radiates into the upper arm, the deltoid insertion should receive an injection of a local anesthetic as well. On the anterolateral aspect of the upper arm,

the deltoid attachment is located in a slight depression. From a mediolateral direction, the needle is advanced until bone contact is made and the injectable is administered in a fan-shaped pattern around the muscle attachment at the deltoid tuberosity of the humerus.

Risks

- Injury to the cephalic vein. Aspiration!
- Unintentional conduction anesthesia of the radial nerve with temporary wrist drop. In the case of galvanic, flashlike sensations during insertion, the needle must be placed more precisely.
- The patient must be informed about the temporary characteristics of anesthesia if numbness or paresthesia is noticed immediately after the injection. Until the regular sensation in the hand is restored, patients should refrain from driving a vehicle.

Concomitant Therapies

- In the case of predominantly inflammatory changes, local cryotherapy is indicated.
- Transverse friction massage at the muscle–tendon junction
- Temporary abducted positioning of the arm
- Phonophoresis
- Stabilization of the shoulder girdle by building up muscle through physical therapy
- Acupuncture, including needling of the periost
- In the case of frozen shoulder, intra-articular saline injection to rupture the capsule, involving manual mobilization and co-treatment of the irritated suprascapular nerve
- In the case of segmental cervical spine dysfunctions, complementing chiropractic treatments
- In the case of calcified humeroscapular periarthritis, extracorporeal shockwave lithotripsy

---

! +++
R 2–3 times a week, up to 12 weeks
PhysApps, FMA, ThE, Acu, Chiro, ESWL

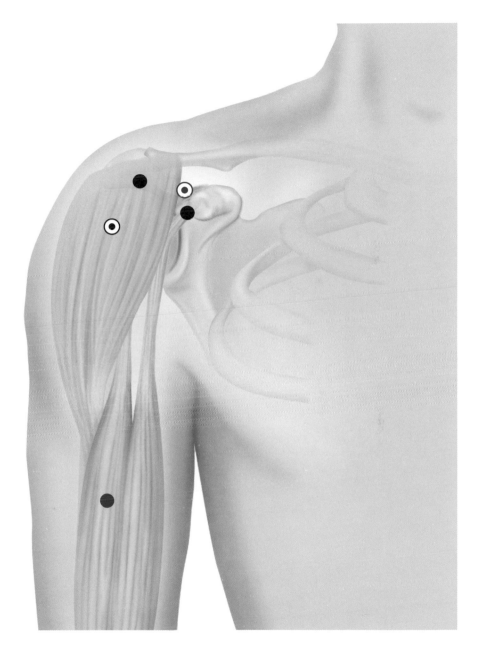

● Primarily indicated injection points

● Complementary point

◉◉ Points of deep injection

Area of pain distribution

Pain in the Area of the Coracoid Process

Indications

- Insertion tendinosis of the pectoralis minor and the coracobrachialis
- Projected pain symptoms to the left of the stomach and the heart
- Right-sided reflex zones of the ascending colon and the liver area

Differential Diagnoses

- Affections of the acromioclavicular joint in terms of arthrosis and blockages
- Inflammatory changes of the subacromial bursa
- Scalene compartment syndrome

Material

- Local anesthetic: 3 mL
- Needle: 0.6 × 30 mm

Technique

- A rough, pressure-sensitive protuberance is located approximately 1–2 cm below the lateral third of the clavicle. This is the fascia-covered coracoid process. The needle is inserted 2–3 cm at the inferior edge of the palpable protuberance.
- The needle is inserted vertically and the injectable is administered in a fan-shaped pattern. It is important to also inject the local anesthetic into the periost of the coracoid process, because the origin site of the short head of the biceps brachii can cause periosteal irritation.

Risks

- The cephalic vein can be injured if the needle is inserted too far medially.
- Aspiration prior to injection can avoid the risk of injecting the local anesthetic into the parallel-running deltoid artery.

Concomitant Therapies

- Treatment with ultrasound in the area of tendon insertions, as well as transverse friction massage
- Iontophoresis
- Acupuncture (LI-15, LU-2, SP-9)

! +++
R 2 times a week, up to 4 weeks
PhysApps, FMA, Acu

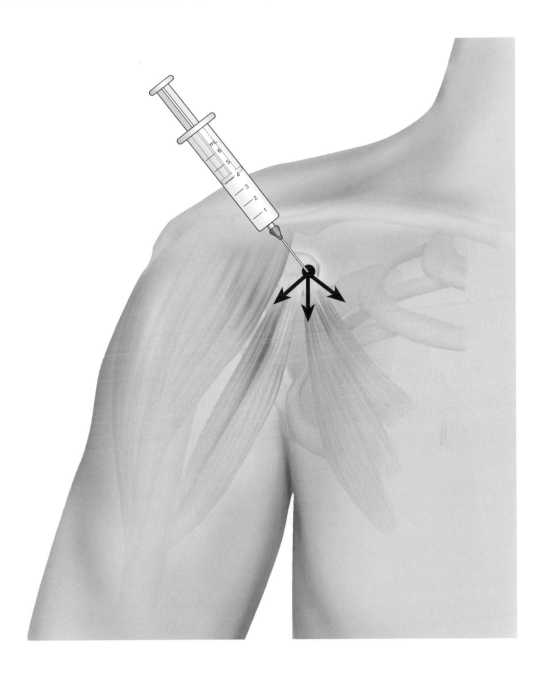

Primarily indicated injection points

Area of pain distribution

Lateral Epicondylitis (Tennis Elbow)

Indications

- Lateral epicondylitis
- Disorders of the radioulnar joint
- Irritation of the anular ligament of the radius
- Myogelosis and insertion tendinosis of the anconeus

Differential Diagnoses

- Shoulder–arm pain due to cervical spine disorders of the C4 segment
- Nerve compartment syndrome (supinator syndrome)
- Herniated disk in the C4/C5 segment
- Free joint bodies
- Osteonecrosis (Hegemann disease, Iselin disease)
- Osteochondritis dissecans of the humeral condyle

Material

- Local anesthetic: 2 mL
- Needle: 0.4 × 20 mm

Technique

- The easily palpable bony protuberance of the condyle of humerus is located. It is generally very pain sensitive.
- Approximately 2 cm distally, the needle is inserted from posterior in the direction of the elbow crease. With use of a fan-shaped pattern, the muscular attachment site is completely flooded with the injectable, particularly the parts close to the bone.

Risks

- If the needle is placed imprecisely and advanced excessively, the radial nerve may be anesthetized. Temporary numbness will result in the area supplied by this nerve, especially on the radial and posterior aspect. Temporary partial paralysis may occur as well.
- If the periost is penetrated and injection takes place in this area, an extremely painful local anesthetic deposit will result between the bone and the periost, which may intensify the initial pain.

Concomitant Therapies

- Functional disorders of the cervical spine segment C4/C5 should bilaterally be ruled out. Beyond that, sensorimotor dysfunctions do not occur. Especially if fingers become numb at night, an affection of the median nerve must be considered.
- In the case of limited mobility and movement disorders in the radioulnar joint, the joint should be treated with manual therapy. If characteristic symptoms of periosteal irritation are present, the patient should apply local cryotherapy, for example, massaging the area with ice cubes. In addition, ultrasound and transverse friction according to Cyriax are recommended.
- Overload relating to work or athletic activities responds well to stretching techniques and additional subcircular taping or supportive bandaging. It is important to gather relevant information about work and athletic activities in the case history. Extracorporeal shockwave treatment is recommended in chronically recurrent cases.

! +++
R 2 times a week, up to 12 weeks
Chiro, PhysApps, FMA, ThE, Orthotech, ESWL

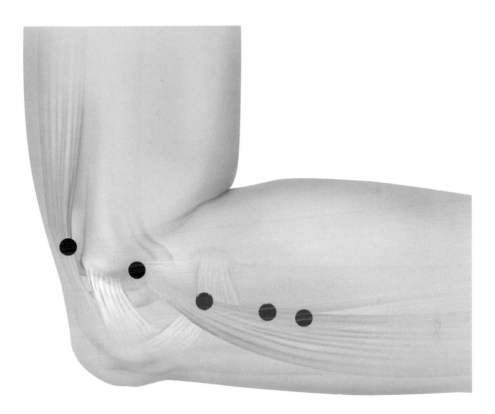

● Primarily indicated injection points

● Complementary point

  Area of pain distribution

Medial Epicondylitis (Golfer's Elbow)

Indications

- Medial epicondylitis
- Pronator teres syndrome
- Arthrosis of the elbow joint
- Periostosis with affection of the ulnar collateral ligament

Differential Diagnoses

- Radicular symptoms of the inferior cervical spine C7/C8
- Cubital tunnel syndrome
- Free joint bodies

Material

- Local anesthetic: 2 mL
- Needle: 0.4 × 20 mm

Technique

- The "two-wall technique" produces the best results. The first injection site is located directly above the most protruding point of the ulna-humeral epicondyle. The needle is advanced up to the periost, retracted 1 mm, and 0.5 mL of a local anesthetic is injected.
- The other points are arranged in the shape of an isosceles triangle, 2 cm distal, deviating slightly in the medial and posterior direction. The fourth point completes an isosceles trapezium and is located a further 2 cm distally on a straight line that comes from the first point and divides the distance between the second and third points in half. The points are located above the pronator teres, flexor carpi radialis, and palmaris longus. The needle is inserted vertically and advanced 1 cm. Each site receives 0.5 mL of a local anesthetic.

Risks

- If the injection takes place posterior to the ulnar epicondyle, the ulnar nerve is anesthetized.
- If the needle is inserted too far proximally at the medial injection site, the injectable may be administered into the ulnar artery.
- At the distal injection sites, unintentional injections into the basilic vein may occur; therefore, aspiration prior to injection is required.

Concomitant Therapies

- Transverse friction massage according to Cyriax, local cryotherapy, and transcutaneous application of anti-inflammatories
- Changes in workload and athletic activities, if applicable
- Phonophoresis
- Acupuncture along the heart and large intestine channels (HT-3, LI-11)

! ++
R 2 times a week, up to 4 weeks
FMA, PhysApps, Acu, Med

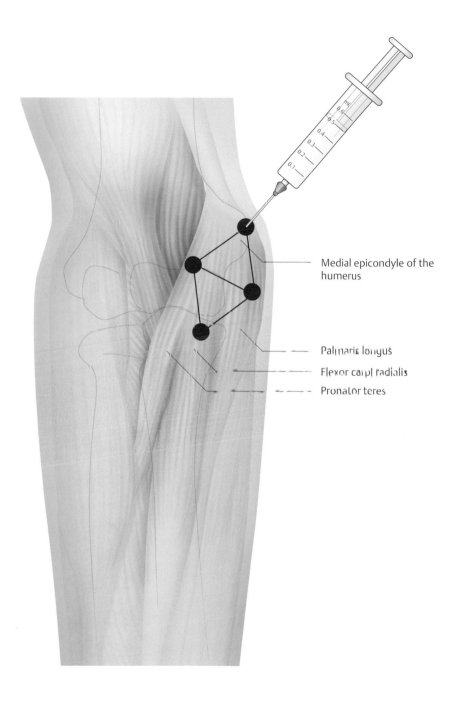

Medial epicondyle of the
humerus

Palmaris longus

Flexor carpi radialis

Pronator teres

● Primarily indicated injection points

  Area of pain distribution

■ Therapy through Muscles, Tendons, and Ligaments

Deltoid

Indications

- Characteristic pain projected in the attachment area of the deltoid, which is located at the deltoid tuberosity on the lateral aspect of the upper arm
- Adjuvant treatment for rotator cuff injuries

Differential Diagnoses

- Affections of the teres minor
- Pain projections in the case of pulmonary affections
- Vascular compartment syndromes, especially scalenus compartment syndromes

Material

- Local anesthetic: 3–5 mL
- Needle: 0.6 × 60 mm

Technique

- The main infiltration sites are located in the area of the deltoid insertion at the lateral aspect of the upper arm. The distinct sensitivity to pressure can be found in this tapering muscle part. The needle is inserted vertically until bone contact is made. The injection includes the periost. The second insertion takes place 1 cm superomedially to the first site. The needle is advanced again until bone contact is made. The third insertion takes place in the same manner, 1.5 cm posterosuperiorly. Each site receives 0.5–1 mL of a local anesthetic.
- Additional injection sites include painful points along the entire deltoid. They can usually be identified as indurated areas within the muscle. With use of the two-finger technique, the distinct pain area receives 0.5 mL of a local anesthetic, 1.5–2 cm deep.

Risks

- Along the anterior border of the deltoid, one may unintentionally inject the local anesthetic into the cephalic vein; therefore, aspiration is necessary prior to injection.
- On the posterior border of the muscle, the local anesthetic may be unintentionally injected into the superior lateral brachial cutaneous nerve of the axillary nerve, which causes temporary numbness in the posterior and lateral aspect of the deltoid. The patient must therefore be informed about possible changes in sensitivity.

Concomitant Therapies

- Local cryotherapy at the deltoid attachment
- Ultrasound in the form of phonophoresis
- Transcutaneous electrical nerve stimulation above the painful areas
- Depending on the stage, physical therapy in the case of rotator cuff injuries
- Medical exercise therapy

! ++
R 2–3 times a week, up to 4 weeks
PhysApps, TENS, ThE, MET

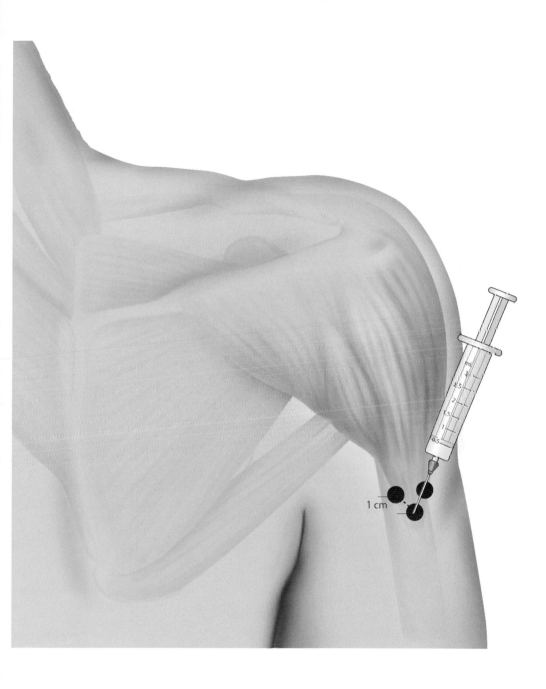

● Primarily indicated injection points

　Area of pain distribution

1 cm

Rhomboid

Indications

- Pain along the superior thoracic spine
- Pain along the medial edge of the shoulder blade

Differential Diagnoses

- Left-sided affections of the posterior myocardial wall
- Affections of the kidneys and the superior urinary tract
- Costovertebral joint dysfunctions

Material

- Local anesthetic: 0.5 mL
- Needle: 0.6 × 30 mm

Technique

- The major and minor rhomboids originate between the first and fifth thoracic vertebra and travel in a transverse-lateral direction to the medial edge of the scapula. The most effective insertion sites are located approximately 2 finger widths medial to the palpable bony edge of the scapula. This is where a distinct, painfully indurated area of the muscle group can be found.
- Beginning at the level of the superior tip of the scapula, needle insertions take place vertically every 3 cm, the needle is advanced 1 cm, and 0.5–1 mL of a local anesthetic is injected.

Risks

- If the needle is advanced excessively, pleura and lungs may be injured; therefore, observe the insertion depth.

Concomitant Therapies

- Local, moist heat application
- Mobilization of the scapula and the scapulo-thoracic gliding plane using manual therapy
- Patients learn to massage the area themselves, for example, using a tennis ball or a porcupine massage ball.
- Brush massage to the muscle group
- Back affusion and hot jet blitz to the back according to Kneipp
- Local application with arnica and camphor
- Local cupping

! +++
R 1–2 times a week, up to 6 weeks
MM, PhysApps, MA, Med

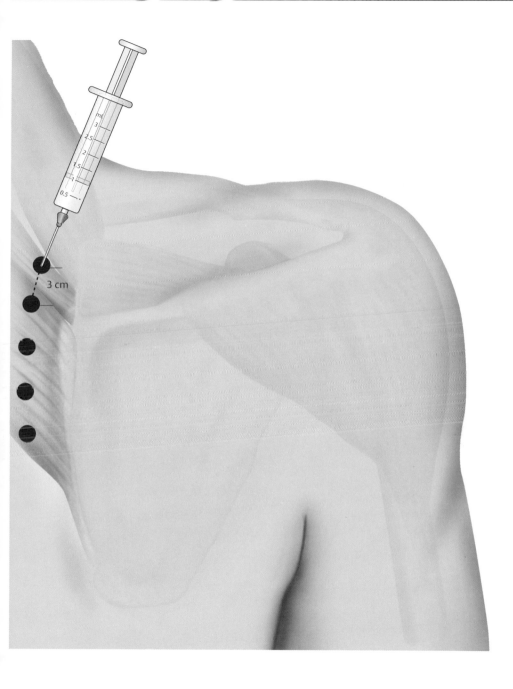

3 cm

● Primarily indicated injection points

  Area of pain distribution

Supraspinatus

Indications

- Humeroscapular periarthritis, tendinopathy, general, calcifying, and fibrotic
- Subacromial impingement
- Adjuvant treatment in the case of degenerative conditions of the rotator cuff
- Adjuvant treatment for fractures of the greater tubercle
- Omarthrosis

Differential Diagnoses

- Referred compartment syndrome of the suprascapular nerve
- Inflammatory changes of the glenohumeral joint
- Left-sided cardiac disorders
- Affections of the acromioclavicular joint

Material

- Local anesthetic: 2 mL
- Needle: 0.6 × 60 mm

Technique

- Subacromially, the posterolateral injection techniques are preferred. Beginning with the palpation of the posterior edge of the acromion, palpation moves laterally along the inferior edge of the acromion. The needle is inserted anteromedially at the inferior edge of the acromion's most lateral aspect. The coracoid process serves for orientation in regard to the direction of insertion.
- The needle is advanced 3 cm. Following aspiration, 1–1.5 mL of a local anesthetic is administered. After the needle has been retracted 1 cm, aspiration is repeated and the remaining local anesthetic is injected.
- Additional injection sites are located in the area of the muscle belly. Coming from a posterior direction, one palpates the scapular crest. Superior to the scapular crest, a wedge-shaped part of the muscle belly is found. In its center, 2–4 additional injections of 0.5 mL each may be administered 3 cm deep.

Risks

- Unintentional intra-articular injection, especially if the needle is inserted too far posteriorly
- Injections into the suprascapular artery can be avoided through prior aspiration.

Concomitant Therapies

- Ultrasound treatment in the area of the tendon attachment of the supraspinatus
- Subacromial glide mobilization using manual therapy
- Transverse friction massage over the tendon attachment of the supraspinatus
- Frequently, concomitant blocks in the C5/C6 segment require manual therapy treatments.
- Application of a cantharis plaster at the attachment site of the supraspinatus is recommended.

! +++
R up to 3 times a week, up to 12 weeks
PhysApps, FMA, Chiro, Med

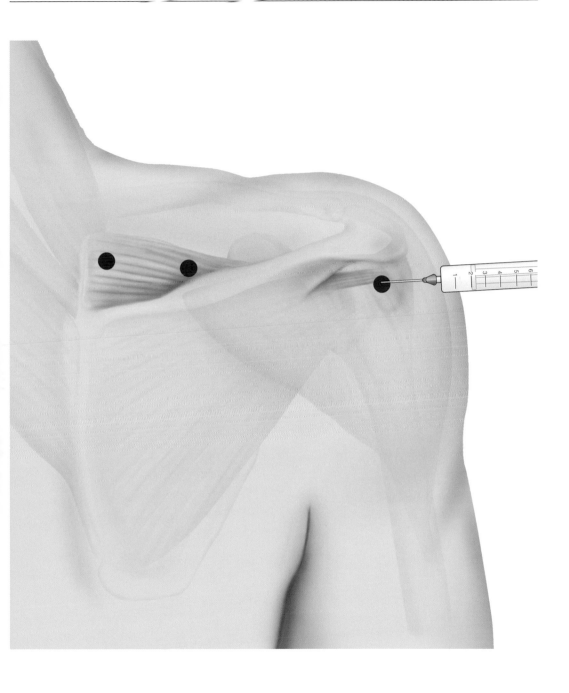

⬤ Primarily indicated injection points

▢ Area of pain distribution

Infraspinatus

Indications

- Myogeloses and pain syndromes of the infraspinatus
- Fibrous shoulder stiffness
- Omarthrosis

Differential Diagnoses

- Referred pain syndromes in duodenal disorders
- Projected pain in the case of subscapularis indurations

Material

- Local anesthetic: 3 mL
- Needle: 0.6 × 60 mm

Technique

- The palpable bony ledge of the scapular crest is located.
- Two to 3 injection sites are located 2 finger widths from the medial scapular edge. The needle is advanced 1 cm and 0.5 mL of a local anesthetic is administered to each site.
- At the attachment site of the greater tubercle of humerus, as well as 1 finger width posteriorly, inferior to the acromion, additional secondary injection sites are found. There, the needle is inserted vertically, advanced 2 cm, and 0.5 mL of a local anesthetic is injected at each site.

Risks

- None

Concomitant Therapies

- Postisometric relaxation of the supraspinatus (tightening in terms of external rotation of the upper arm against resistance followed by passive internal rotation mobilization)
- Friction massage with a small massage stick
- Local moxibustion of the painful areas is effective but is perceived as intolerably painful by many patients.
- Physical therapy
- Medical exercise therapy

! +++
R 2 times a week, up to 4 weeks
PIR, FMA, MET, ThE

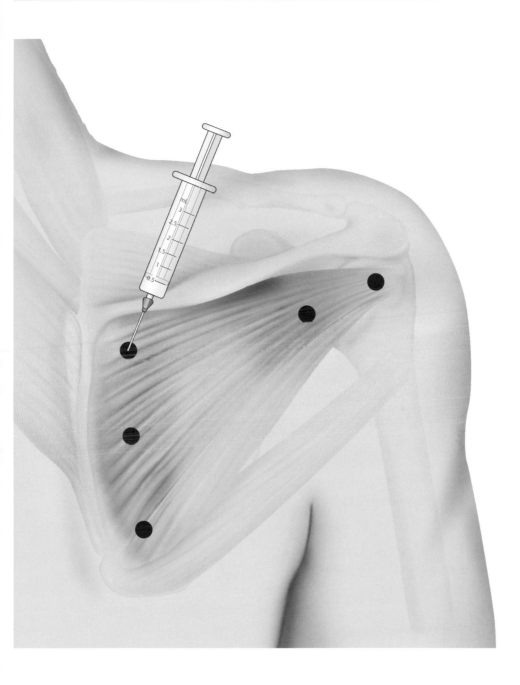

● Primarily indicated injection points

  Area of pain distribution

Biceps Brachii

Indications

- Insertion tendinosis of the biceps brachii at the superior attachment and myositis at the inferior myotendinous junction
- Pain patterns after rupturing of the long biceps tendon

Differential Diagnosis

- Radicular symptoms, especially with C5/C6 affection
- Compartment syndrome of the axillary neurovascular bundle

Material

- Local anesthetic: 3 mL
- Needle: 0.6 × 60 mm

Technique

- The coracoid process is located in the area of the anterior armpit. It is easily palpable and usually sensitive to pressure. The first injection takes place lateral to the lower edge of the coracoid process. The needle is inserted vertically, advanced 2 cm, and 0.5 mL of a local anesthetic is injected.
- The second insertion site is located in the area of the proximal humerus. The anterior aspects of the bicipital groove can be located through slight internal/external rotation of the arm. Here, the needle is inserted and advanced until bone contact is made. After the needle has been retracted 1–2 mm, 0.5 mL of a local anesthetic is injected. The middle injection sites are located at the central muscle belly of the biceps brachii. At a depth of 1.5 cm, 0.5 mL of a local anesthetic is administered to the medial and to the lateral muscle belly.
- The distal injections site is located in the area of the tapered myotendinous junction. Still on the muscular aspect, a distinct pressure-sensitive painful area of approximately finger-tip size can be found. Here, the needle is inserted vertically, advanced 1 cm, and 1 mL of a local anesthetic is injected.

Risks

- Unintentional injection into the cephalic vein is possible at the medial and distal injection sites. There are no further risks if the depth of insertion is observed.

Concomitant Therapies

- Proximally, phonophoresis at the tendinoperiosteal junction
- Continuous tightening exercises for the muscle
- Cryogenic friction massage at the distal myotendinous junction

! +
R 2 times a week, up to 4 weeks
PhysApps, FMA, MET

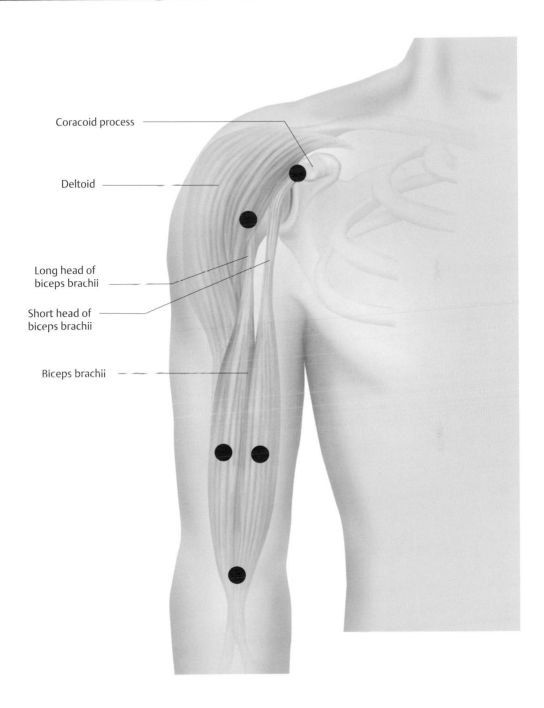

Coracoid process

Deltoid

Long head of
biceps brachii

Short head of
biceps brachii

Biceps brachii

Primarily indicated injection points

Area of pain distribution

Triceps Brachii

Indications

- Generally, nonspecific pain in the area of the posterior upper arm
- In the elbow area, radiating pain that is difficult to localize and is frequently misdiagnosed as tennis elbow. Extension against resistance and distinct sensitivity to pressure proximal to the olecranon are an indication.
- Adjuvant treatment in the case of chronic bursitis of the olecranon
- Adjuvant treatment in the case of elbow arthrosis

Differential Diagnoses

- Radicular pain radiating from T 1
- Costovertebral joint blockage at the cervicothoracic junction

Material

- Local anesthetic: 2–4 mL
- Needle: 0.4 × 20 mm

Technique

- The distal attachment of the triceps brachii is fixed between the thumb and the index finger while the patient's elbow is slightly flexed. Directly proximal to the palpable olecranon, the needle is inserted and advanced 0.5 cm, and 0.5 mL of a local anesthetic is injected.
- The second injection site is located 4 cm superior to the first site, on the posterior median line of the triceps brachii. This is the myotendinous junction. The needle is advanced 0.5 cm and 0.5–1 mL of a local anesthetic is injected.
- The proximal injection sites are located a further 3 cm proximal to the second site, each deviating 1 cm, medially and laterally, above the muscle bellies of the long head and the lateral head of the triceps brachii. The needle is advanced 1 cm and 0.5 mL of a local anesthetic is injected.

Concomitant Therapies

- Supracondylar support tape
- Traction and extension as part of physical therapy
- Transverse friction massage

! ++
R 2 times a week, up to 6 weeks
ThE, FMA, Orthotech

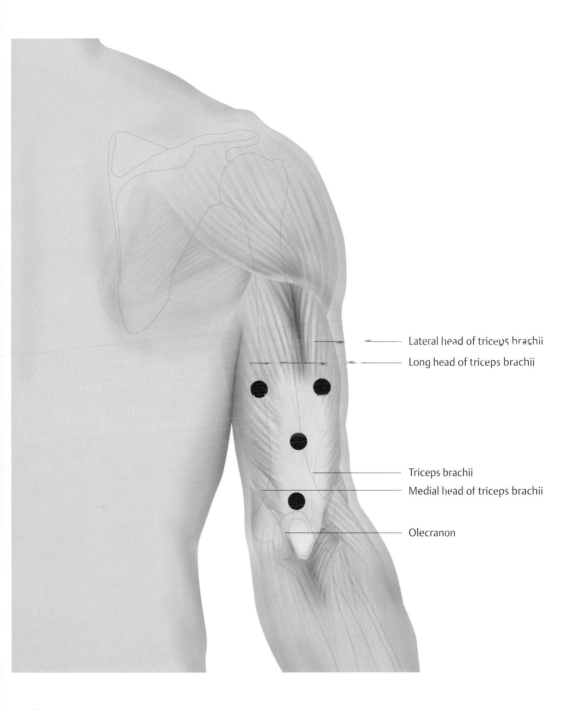

Lateral head of triceps brachii

Long head of triceps brachii

Triceps brachii

Medial head of triceps brachii

Olecranon

Primarily indicated injection points

Area of pain distribution

Supinator

Indications

- Supinator compartment syndrome
- Humeroulnar arthroses
- Inflammatory elbow affections

Differential Diagnoses

- Epicondylitis
- Affections of the radial collateral ligament, radicular symptoms of the C8 segment

Material

- Local anesthetic: 2 mL
- Needle: 0.6 × 60 mm

Technique

- With the patient's elbow supinated and slightly flexed, the needle is inserted 2 cm distally to the elbow crease. The lateral muscle belly is fixed between the thumb and the index finger. The needle is advanced until bone contact is made. After the needle has been retracted 0.5 cm, 1–2 mL of a local anesthetic is injected.

Risks

- Inserting the needle too far distally may injure the radial artery.
- Unintentional conduction anesthesia of the superficial branch of the radial nerve may occur if prior bone contact is not made.

Concomitant Therapies

- Mobilization of the humeroradial joint using manual therapy
- Transverse friction massage in terms of cryogenic friction massage with little massage sticks

! ++
R 2 times a week, up to 6 weeks
MM, FMA

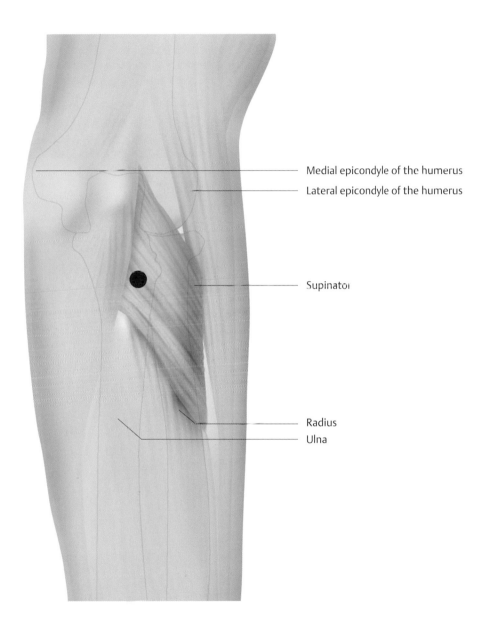

Medial epicondyle of the humerus

Lateral epicondyle of the humerus

Supinator

Radius

Ulna

● Primarily indicated injection points

Area of pain distribution

Trigger Finger

Indications

- Characteristic triggering phenomenon usually of the second, third, and fourth fingers. The painful extension block is located at the metacarpophalangeal joint.

Differential Diagnoses

- None, if symptoms are characteristic

Material

- Local anesthetic: 1 mL
- Needle: 0.4 × 20 mm

Technique

- The nodular and fusiform thickening of the flexor tendon is usually easy to palpate.
- After the thickened area has been located, the needle is inserted tangentially, at a shallow angle, and the injectable is administered paratendinously, 0.5 mL to the right and to the left of the tendon into the tendon sheath.

Risks

- Anesthesia of the common palmar digital nerves.
- Inserting the needle too far proximally may result in injection of local anesthetic into the superficial palmar arch; therefore, aspiration is necessary prior to injection.

Concomitant Therapies

- Regular functional therapy in terms of mud treatment, temporary application of a posterior forearm splint
- One-time application of a low-dose corticosteroid, if applicable
- In persistent cases, surgical treatment

! +
R once a week, up to 4 weeks
ThE, Orthotech, Med

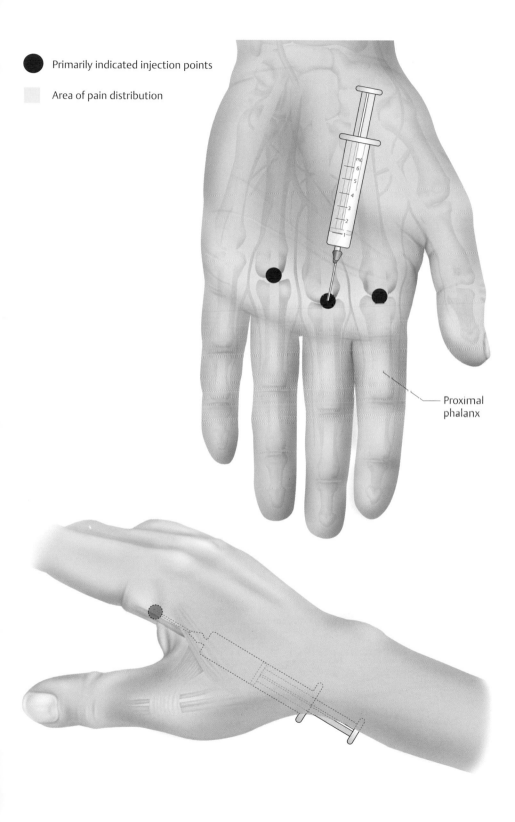

● Primarily indicated injection points

▢ Area of pain distribution

Proximal phalanx

Pain in the Area of the Radial Styloid Process

Indications

- Distinct insertion tendinosis of the extensor carpi radialis and the flexor carpi radialis
- Arthroses of the wrist

Differential Diagnoses

- De Quervain tenosynovitis (Finkelstein test results negative)
- Insertion tendinitis of the brachioradialis

Material

- Local anesthetic: 0.5–1 mL
- Needle: 0.4 × 20 mm

Technique

- The injection site is located directly above the pressure-sensitive spot at the tip of the styloid process.
- The needle is inserted vertically and advanced until bone contact is made. Small quantities of the injectable are administered in a fan-shaped pattern.

Risks

- Puncturing of the radial artery; therefore, aspiration and contact of the needle with bone are necessary prior to injection.

Concomitant Therapies

- Cryotherapy, supportive taping, immobilization through a forearm splint
- Periosteal massage

! ++
R 2 times a week, up to 6 weeks
PhysApps, Orthotech, MA, Med

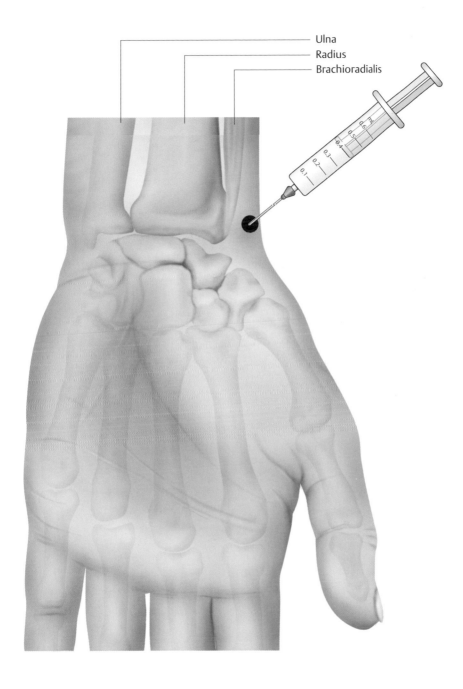

Ulna
Radius
Brachioradialis

● Primarily indicated injection points

  Area of pain distribution

Pain in the Area of the Ulnar Styloid Process

Indications

- Distinct insertion tendinosis of the extensor carpi ulnaris and the flexor carpi ulnaris
- Conditions resulting from forearm and wrist fractures
- Pain resulting from necrosis of carpal bones
- Arthroses of the wrist

Differential Diagnoses

- Compression syndrome in the area of the Guyon canal (ulnar canal)

Material

- Local anesthetic: 0.5–1 mL
- Needle: 0.4 × 20 mm

Technique

- The needle is inserted directly above the painful spot and advanced until bone contact is made.
- Small quantities of the injectable are administered in a fan-shaped pattern around the center of pain.

Risks

- If the needle is injected too far palmarly, the ulnar nerve may be anesthetized and the ulnar artery punctured. This is avoided by advancing the needle tip right up to the bone.

Concomitant Therapies

- Repeated cryotherapy
- Supportive taping proximally, cantharis plaster
- Periosteal massage

! ++
R 2 times a week, up to 6 weeks
PhysApps, Orthotech, MA, Med

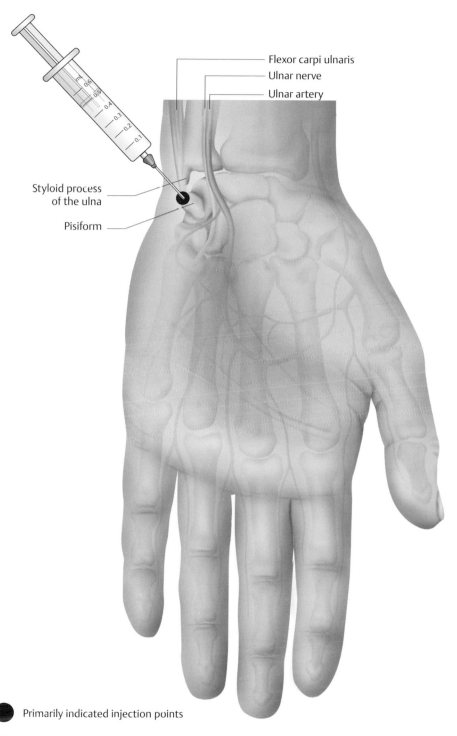

Flexor carpi ulnaris

Ulnar nerve

Ulnar artery

Styloid process
of the ulna

Pisiform

● Primarily indicated injection points

Area of pain distribution

Tenosynovitis Stenosans

Indications

- Irritation of the tendon sheath in the area of the abductor pollicis and the extensor pollicis
- De Quervain tenosynovitis
- Arthralgia of the proximal wrist
- Adjuvant treatment in terms of injection acupuncture on the large intestine channel (LI-5), as well as a point for tonification on the lung channel (LU-9)

Differential Diagnoses

- Arthritis of the wrist
- Carpal blockage
- Necrosis of the lunate bone and pseudoarthrosis following fracture of the navicular bone
- Radiating pain in terms of a distal interference field originating in changes within the scalenus and the brachioradialis

Material

- Local anesthetic: 3 mL
- Needle: 0.4 × 20 mm

Technique

- The distal injection site is located at the junction of the first metacarpal and the proximal phalanx. This is where the extensor pollicis brevis attaches. The bony protuberance is very prominent when the thumb is flexed. The course of the tendon can be assessed while the thumb is abducted against resistance. The needle is advanced until bone contact is made and 0.5 mL of the injectable is administered.
- The proximal injection site is located while the thumb is abducted. A depression can be found on the wrist, between the long and the short thumb abductor. A local anesthetic is injected into the noticeably stronger strand in the first extensor tendon compartment. The retinaculum encompasses the wrist like a bracelet. With the needle pointing toward the wrist, it is inserted below the retinaculum into both sides of the protruding tendon. Additional injections of the local anesthetic into the extensor pollicis longus tendon take place while passing the retinaculum and, 1 cm proximally, into the myotendinous

junction of the extensor pollicis brevis. Here, the needle may be advanced until bone contact is made and it is retracted 2–3 mm prior to injection.

Risks

- Injury of the radial artery; therefore, prior aspiration is vital. Never administer the injectable if blood is aspirated.
- Anesthesia of the superficial branch of the radial nerve with numbness of the area of the thumb.
- An infection of the joint may result from unintentional intra-articular injection if the proper hygiene protocol is ignored; therefore, careful attention to asepsis is required.

Concomitant Therapies

- Additional transcutaneous nerve stimulation (transcutaneous electrical nerve stimulation/ TENS)
- Local cryotherapy with an anti-inflammatory occlusive or supportive bandage, short-termed splinting
- Postisometric relaxation technique for the extensor pollicis longus and extensor pollicis brevis
- Surgical treatment, if necessary

! +++
R 2–3 times a week, up to 6 weeks
TENS, Med, Orthotech, PIR, ThE, Surg

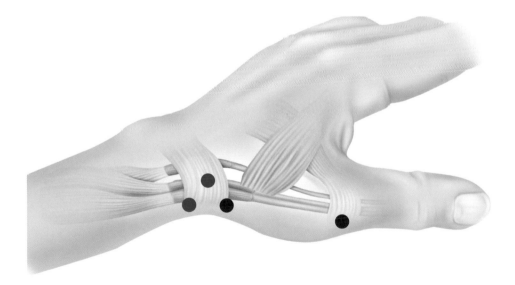

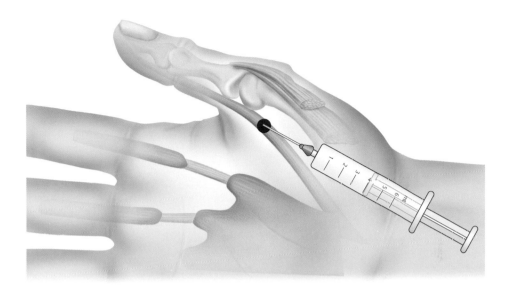 Primarily indicated injection points

Complementary point

■ Therapy through Nerves

Suprascapular Nerve

Indications

- Chronic pain syndromes of the shoulder joint, the acromioclavicular joint, and the subacromial area that are resistant to therapy
- Compartment syndrome of the suprascapular nerve

Differential Diagnoses

- Radicular C4/C5 syndromes
- Scalenus compartment syndrome
- Inflammatory changes within the acromioclavicular joint
- Inflammation of the subacromial bursa

Material

- Local anesthetic: 4 mL
- Needle: 0.8 × 80 mm

Technique

- While the patient is seated with arms folded in front of the chest, a line is drawn along the scapular crest. Parallel to the spinous processes, a vertical line is drawn that halves the first line. The insertion site is located 2 cm lateral and superior to the intersection. The angle of the needle during insertion points slightly mediocaudally.
- The needle is advanced 5–7 cm. All the way to the notch, the bone can be carefully sought with the tip of the needle.

Risks

- Rare but possible is the occurrence of a pneumothorax if the needle is advanced excessively; therefore, the depth of needle insertion must be observed.
- Caution: If the subscapular nerve is completely anesthetized, the supraspinatus and infraspinatus fail to function. For the duration of the local anesthesia, this leads to partial paralysis in regard to abduction and external rotation.

Concomitant Therapies

- Especially in the case of frozen shoulder, the shoulder should be mobilized when anesthesia takes effect.
- In the case of chronic neuralgia, vitamin B combination treatment
- Transcutaneous electrical nerve stimulation
- Manual mobilization

!+++
R initially daily, later 2 times a week, up to 12 weeks
ThE, Med, MM, TENS

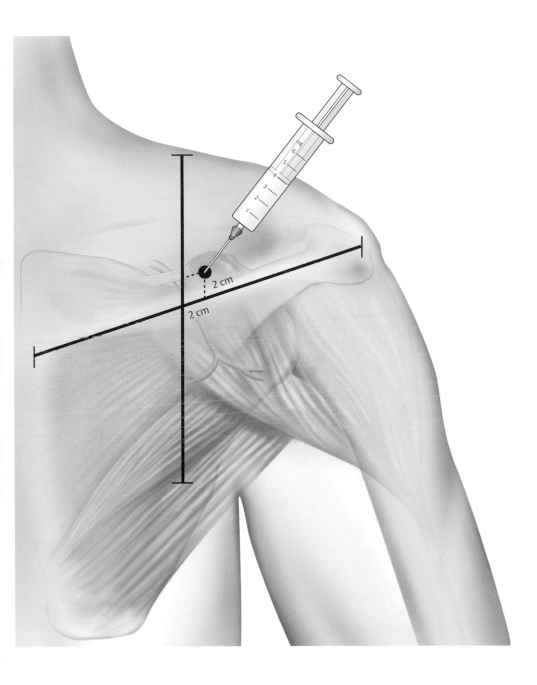

2 cm

2 cm

● Primarily indicated injection points

   Area of pain distribution

Median Nerve

Indications

- Carpal tunnel syndrome

Differential Diagnoses

- Irritation of the flexor tendon
- Necrosis of the lunate bone
- Arthroses of the wrist
- Radicular C5/C6 syndromes

Material

- Local anesthetic: 2 mL
- Needle: 0.4 × 20 mm

Technique

- The needle is inserted from the palmar wrist fold toward the fingers. The insertion site is ulnar to the well-visible tendon of the palmaris longus.
- The needle is inserted transversely at a very shallow angle and is advanced relatively far, 1–1.5 cm. Paresthesias are frequently triggered during the injection. A local anesthetic (1–2 mL) is administered.

Risks

- None, if the standard protocol is observed

Concomitant Therapies

- Application of a posterior forearm splint with the arm in the neutral position
- Administration of vitamin B supplements
- Attempt at systemic dehydration
- In the case of persistence, surgical treatment, such as neurolysis, and division of the transverse carpal ligament

! +++
R 1–2 times a week, up to 6 months
Orthotech, Med, Surg

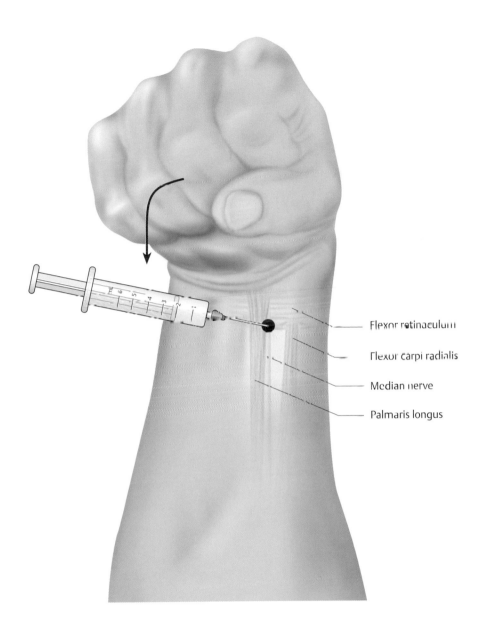

Flexor retinaculum

Flexor carpi radialis

Median nerve

Palmaris longus

● Primarily indicated injection points

▢ Area of pain distribution

■ Intra-articular Therapy

Shoulder Joint (Glenohumeral Joint)

Indications

- Idiopathic or posttraumatic arthritis
- Capsulitis
- Frozen shoulder

Material

- Local anesthetic: 10 mL
- Needle: 0.9 × 70 mm

Technique

- The needle is inserted from the posterior aspect of the shoulder. To locate the site, the patient is seated with the arm hanging down, bent at the elbow, and the forearm is held in front of the abdomen. The thumb of the practitioner's free hand palpates posteriorly the edge of the acromial angle. The index finger palpates anteriorly the coracoid process and remains on its tip.
- The insertion takes place 1 cm inferior to the thumb mark, with the needle tip pointing toward the index finger.
- The injection can be done smoothly and without pressure if the needle is inserted correctly into the intra-articular space. Increased pressure during the injection indicates misplacement of the needle.

Risks

- Injection into the axillary artery and anesthesia of the axillary plexus if the needle is inserted too deep and too far medially. It is therefore important to insert the needle toward the index finger that rests on the tip of the coracoid process and to remember to perform aspiration prior to injection.

Concomitant Therapies

- Manual traction mobilization
- Cryotherapy
- Positioning of the arm in abduction
- Administration of nonsteroidal antirheumatic agents with systemic effect

! +++
R 1–2 times a week
PhysApps, ThE

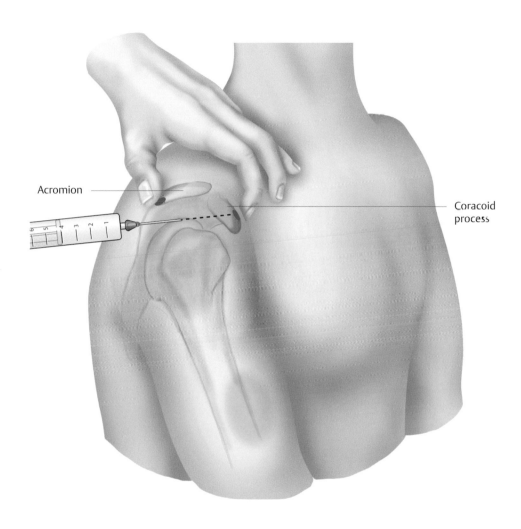

Acromion

Coracoid process

Elbow Joint (Humeroradial/Humeroulnar Joint)

Indications

- Arthritis
- Degenerative changes
- Partial stiffness of the elbow joint

Differential Diagnoses

- Lateral epicondylitis
- Supinator compartment syndrome
- Free joint bodies

Material

- Local anesthetic: 2 mL
- Needle: 0.6 × 30 mm

Technique

- The patient is seated with the elbow flexed at a 90° angle. The forearm is 90° pronated and rests on a support. The lateral head of the radius is palpated. The finding is confirmed by passively pronating and supinating the forearm beneath the palpating finger, which can feel the rotating head of the radius.
- Coming from the lateral direction, one inserts the needle vertically and advances it toward the medial epicondyle of the humerus.
- When the needle is being advanced, resistance is felt during penetration of the joint capsule. Smooth injection, without pressure, indicates the correct intra-articular position of the needle.

Risks

- None

Concomitant Therapies

- Manual mobilization
- Local cryotherapy
- Short-term immobilization through the application of a posterior upper arm/forearm splint

! ++
R once a week
PhysApps, TENS, Orthotech

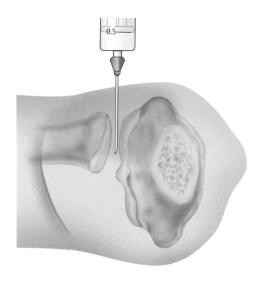

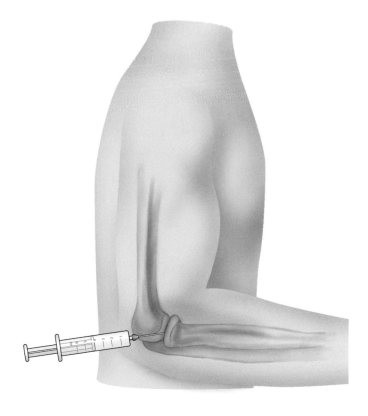

Wrist (Radiocarpal Joint)

Indications

* Degenerative traumatic or rheumatoid arthritis

Differential Diagnoses

* Arthrosis or necrosis of the lunate bone
* Irritation of the distal radioulnar joint

Material

* Local anesthetic: 2 mL
* Needle: 0.6 × 30 mm

Technique

* The patient is seated with the forearm pronated. The hand is placed on a pillow in 30° flexion.
* The joint line is palpated and marked radially and ulnarly. The two marks are connected with an auxiliary line. The hand is actively extended, which allows the tendon of the extensor carpi radialis to be identified.
* The insertion site is located on the ulnar side, next to the extensor carpi, at the level of the auxiliary line on the wrist. The direction of needle insertion is 15° toward the elbow. After the joint capsule has been penetrated, the local anesthetic can be smoothly administered.

Risks

* The needle is located intracapsular; therefore, never inject the local anesthetic by force.

Concomitant Therapy

* Temporary immobilization through application of a palmar forearm/hand splint
* Cryotherapy
* Application of a topical anti-inflammatory and administration of nonsteroidal antirheumatic agents with systemic effect

! ++
R once a week
Orthotech, Cryo

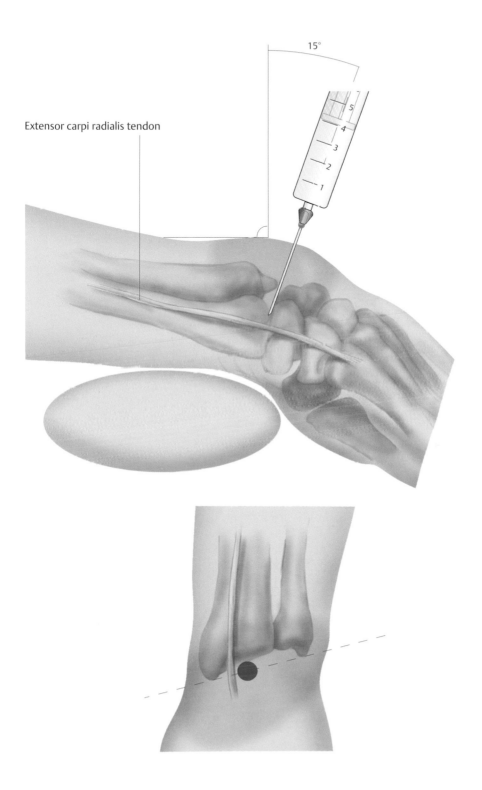

Extensor carpi radialis tendon

15°

Rhizarthrosis and Pain Syndromes of the Thumb Saddle Joint

Indications

- Rhizarthrosis, pain syndromes with affection of the adductor pollicis
- Affections of the thumb saddle joint

Differential Diagnoses

- Irritations of the superficial radial nerve
- Different forms of tenosynovitis, for example, De Quervain disease

Material

- Local anesthetic: 2 mL
- Needle: 0.4 × 20 mm

Technique

- The needle is inserted vertically, with the patient's thumb slightly abducted. The insertion site is ulnar to the tendon of the extensor pollicis longus, between the first metacarpal and the trapezium bone. To locate the narrow joint line, the needle tip should feel its way into the joint capsule. After penetrating the joint capsule, the needle drops a few millimeters into the joint. A local anesthetic (0.2–0.5 mL) can be administered without applying increased plunger pressure.
- The second insertion site is located above the most voluminous area of the adductor pollicis belly. During end-range adduction of the thumb, the needle is inserted from posterior into the crest of the protruding adductor pollicis.
- Additional anesthesia of the superficial branch of the radial nerve is recommended in the case of painful chronic disorders. This block is placed on the palmar aspect of the wrist crease. After the pulse of the radial artery has been palpated, the needle is inserted a few millimeters radially to the pulse and advanced 0.5–1 cm. Then, 0.5 mL of a local anesthetic is injected.

Risks

- If the needle is advanced excessively into the thumb saddle joint, the palmarly running tendon of the flexor carpi radialis may be injured.
- If the needle is inserted too close to the pulse of the radial artery, unintentional injection into the radial artery is possible; therefore, aspiration is vital.

Concomitant Therapies

- Manual therapy in terms of mobilization of the thumb saddle joint applying traction
- Local mud treatment therapy
- Anti-inflammatory, blood-flow-promoting occlusive bandage
- Splinting, if applicable
- Sole baths for the hand

! +++
R once a week, long-term treatment, if necessary
MM, PhysApps, Med, Orthotech

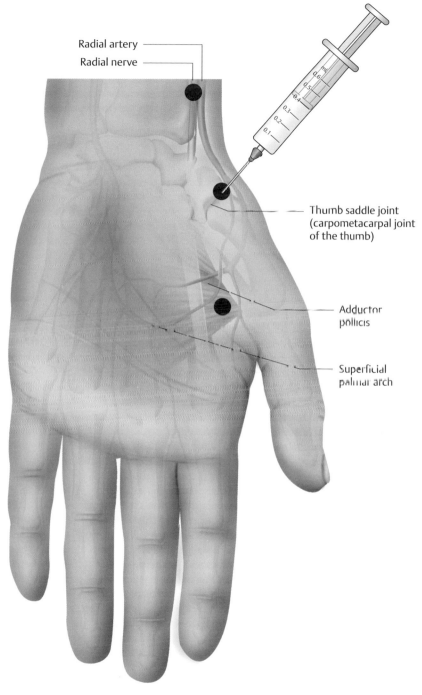

Radial artery

Radial nerve

Thumb saddle joint
(carpometacarpal joint
of the thumb)

Adductor
pollicis

Superficial
palmar arch

● Primarily indicated injection points

Area of pain distribution

5 Thorax and Abdomen

■ Complex Pain

Xiphoid–Sternum–Clavicle Triangle

Indications

- Sternum pain, painful sternoclavicular joint, painful sternoclavicular joint in the case of arthrosis, and conditions following clavicle fracture
- Emphysematous thorax including xiphoid pain

Differential Diagnoses

- Intestinal and mediastinal affections
- Respiratory disorders

Material

- Local anesthetic: 2.5 mL
- Needle: 0.6 × 30 mm

Technique

- The sternoclavicular joint is easily palpable. The clavicle is palpated up to its medial sternal end, where the palpating finger drops into a depression. The joint line can be palpated by moving the arm. The needle is inserted vertically 0.5 cm and 0.5 mL of a local anesthetic is injected.
- This procedure is performed at both sternoclavicular joints and is followed by locating the xiphoid; this bone–cartilage process is usually distinctly pressure sensitive at one spot. The needle is inserted vertically 1 cm (observe the depth of insertion) and 1.5 mL of a local anesthetic is injected.

Risks

- If the needle is inserted excessively deep and the joint line is missed, a pneumothorax may occur at the sternoclavicular joint.
- If the injectable is administered excessively deep at the xiphoid process, abdominal organs may be injured.

Concomitant Therapies

- Mobilization of the sternoclavicular joint using manual therapy
- Postisometric relaxation of the rectus abdominis
- Consistently exercising the levator scapulae
- Stretching treatment for the shortened pectoralis major

! ++
R 2 times a week, up to 8 weeks
MM, ThE, MET

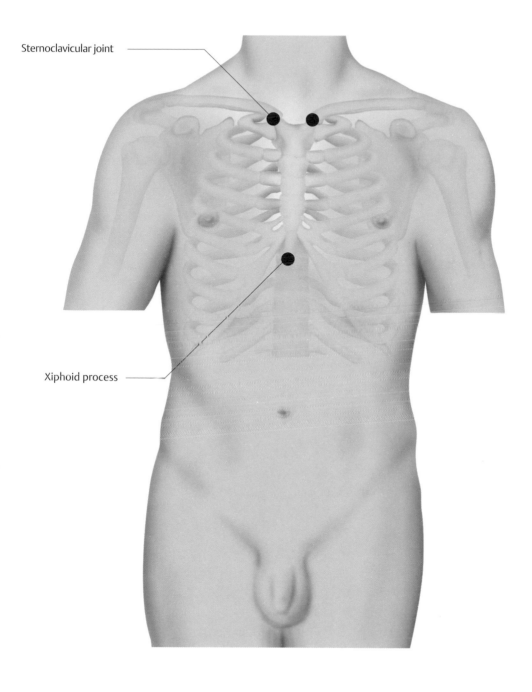

Sternoclavicular joint

Xiphoid process

● Primarily indicated injection points

  Area of pain distribution

Interscapular Pain

Indications

- Interscapular pain
- Thoracic syndrome accompanying obstructive respiratory disorders, for example, bronchial asthma

Differential Diagnoses

- Affections of the pleural dome
- Cardiac disorders

Material

- Local anesthetic: 5 mL
- Needle: 0.6 × 30 mm

Technique

- A vertical line is drawn 3 cm lateral to the spinous processes. Along this line, the needle is inserted vertically every 2 cm.
- At each site, an intracutaneous quaddle containing 0.5 mL of a local anesthetic is set, then the needle is advanced 1 cm and a further 0.5 mL of a local anesthetic is injected. Injections follow the pathway of the bladder meridian.

Risks

- If the needle is advanced excessively, there may be the rare occurrence of a pneumothorax, especially at the vertex of the kyphosis; therefore, the depth of insertion must be observed.

Concomitant Therapies

- Local warm peloid application, combined with mobilization of the subscapularis and lateral traction mobilization
- Relaxation massages, acupuncture treatments
- Hot jet blitz to the back, according to Kneipp
- Chiropractic therapy

! ++
R 3 times a week, up to 8 weeks
PhysApps, ThE, Met, Chiro

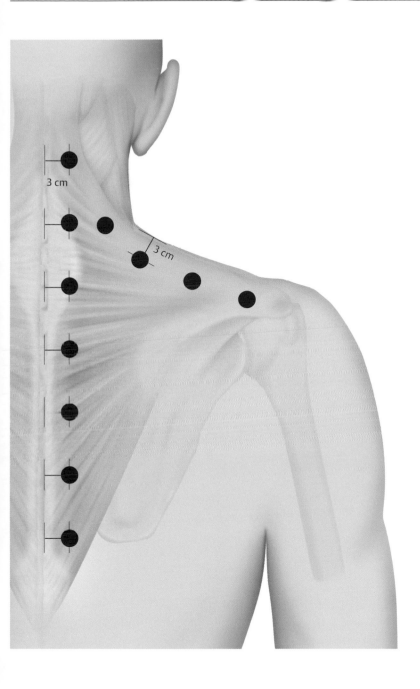

3 cm

3 cm

● Primarily indicated injection points

Area of pain distribution

■ Therapy through Muscles, Tendons, and Ligaments

Pectoralis Major

Indications

- Painful shortening of the pectoralis major accompanied by myotendinous irritation
- Adjuvant treatment in emphysema
- Adjuvant treatment in painful sternocostal joints
- Adjuvant treatment in respiratory disorders

Material

- Local anesthetic: 4 mL
- Needle: 0.6 × 30 mm

Technique

- Beginning at the mamillary line, the injectable is administered intramuscularly every 3 cm along a line that curves slightly laterally. Frequently, distinct pressure-sensitive myogeloses are found on that line. These points are fixed with the two-finger technique, the needle is inserted vertically 1 cm, and 1 mL of the injectable is administered.
- In addition, a local anesthetic is always injected into the attachment at the upper arm. The inferior border of the pectoralis major is traced to the humerus. The needle is inserted 1 cm superiorly toward the bone until bone contact is made. After the needle has been retracted 1–2 mm, 1 mL of a local anesthetic is injected.

Risks

- None

Concomitant Therapies

- Especially physical therapy, including stretching and postisometric relaxation of the pectoralis major and pectoralis minor
- Mobilization of the costovertebral joints using manual therapy
- Medical assessment of the workplace or adequate assessment of motion sequences during athletic activities, if applicable
- Friction massage of the pectoralis major

! ++
R 2 times a week, up to 8 weeks
ThE, PIR, MM

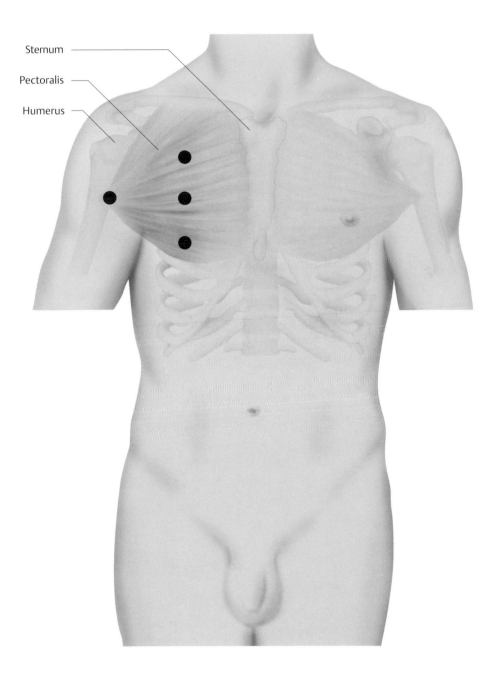

Sternum

Pectoralis

Humerus

● Primarily indicated injection points

Area of pain distribution

Sternocostalis

Indications

- Diffuse pectoral pain
- Tietze syndrome
- Sternocostal joint dysfunctions
- Pain syndromes following rib fractures

Material

- Local anesthetic: 0.5 mL per sternocostal joint
- Needle: 0.4 × 20 mm

Technique

- Initially, the sternum is palpated. From there, the finger moves laterally to the palpable sternocostal joint. The precise position is confirmed by having the patient inhale and exhale deeply; this allows the physician to palpate the motion within the sternocostal joint. The needle is inserted vertically 0.5 cm and 0.5 mL of a local anesthetic is injected.
- If necessary, the joint line is felt for after the needle tip has made bone contact.

Risks

- If the needle is advanced excessively, the pleura or the left pericardium may be injured; therefore, the depth of insertion must be observed.

Concomitant Therapies

- Mobilization and manipulation of the sternocostal joint using manual therapy
- Acupuncture on the kidney channel, especially KI-22–KI-27, in combination with BL-11–BL-19
- Friction massage of the intercostals, topical anti-inflammatory therapy

! +++
R 1–2 times per week, up to 4 weeks
MM, Acu, FMA, Med

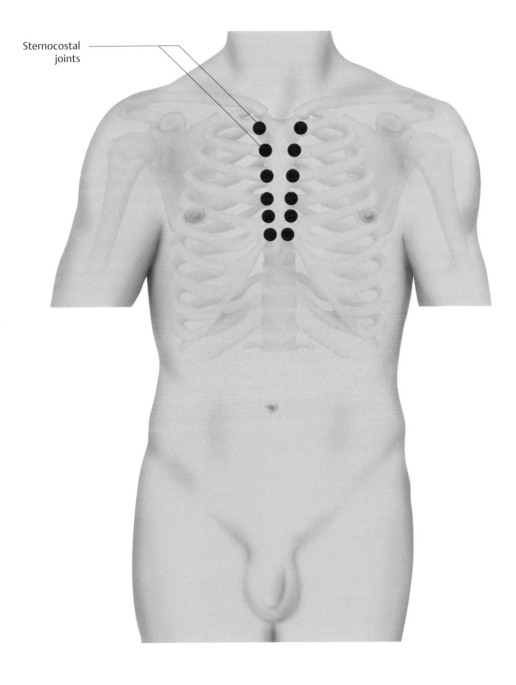

Sternocostal joints

● Primarily indicated injection points

Area of pain distribution

Rectus Abdominis

Indications

- Myotendinous complaints in the muscle area
- Diffuse complaints in the upper abdomen, sub-costally radiating complaints accompanied by back pain
- Adjuvant treatment in small intestine dysfunction

Material

- Local anesthetic: 5 mL
- Needle: 0.6 × 30 mm

Technique

- The proximal row of injections is along the area of the costal triangle and the xiphoid process; here, the needle is inserted vertically 0.5 cm directly subcostal and inferior to the xiphoid process, respectively. Every 2 cm, 0.5 mL of a local anesthetic is injected.
- In the second and third rows, 3 finger widths distally, the injection sites are located 2 cm lateral on both sides of the median line on the bulges of the rectus abdominis. The needle is inserted 1 cm and 0.5 mL of the injectable is administered.
- The distal injection sites are located directly superior to the symphysis, 1 finger width lateral on both sides of the median line. Initially, the superior edge of the symphysis is palpated. The needle is then inserted vertically 2 cm, until bone contact is made. Superior to the bone, the needle is advanced 0.5 cm and 0.5 mL of a local anesthetic is injected per side.

Risks

- If the needle is advanced excessively, the abdominal organs or the bladder may be injured; therefore, the depth of insertion must be observed. The recommended depth of insertion refers to the average Central European; in adipose patients, the individual premuscular adipose tissue must be considered.

Concomitant Therapies

- Warm and moist abdominal poultices
- Vibration massage
- Ultrasound application in the area of the pubic attachment
- Subcostal application of essential mint oil extracts
- Respiratory therapy

! +++
R 2–3 times per week, up to 6 weeks
PhysApps, MA, Med, ThE

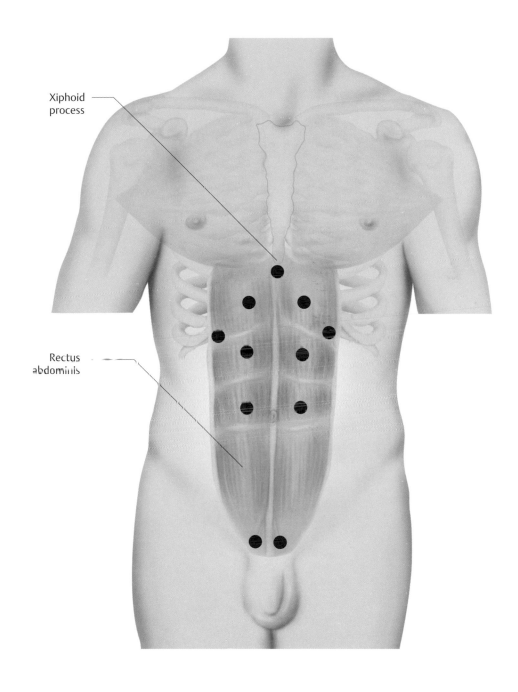

Xiphoid
process

Rectus
abdominis

● Primarily indicated injection points

  Area of pain distribution

Transversus Abdominis

Indications

- Especially subcostal pain, frequently accompanied by chronic respiratory disorders
- Less frequently, pain syndromes due to work-related incorrect posture

Differential diagnoses

- Basal pulmonary affections

Material

- Local anesthetic: 5 mL
- Needle: 0.6 × 30 mm

Technique

- Below the easily palpable costal arch, bilateral insertions are made semicircularly toward the palpable rib until bone contact is made. After the needle has been retracted 2–3 mm, 0.5 mL of the local anesthetic is injected; this is repeated bilaterally every 3 cm.
- In addition, the same injection procedure should be repeated along the ventral iliac crest. The needle is advanced to the iliac crest and retracted 2–3 mm. Then, 0.5 mL of a local anesthetic is injected.

Concomitant Therapies

- Especially subcostal phonophoretic applications
- Local warm peloid application and body wraps
- Respiratory therapy
- Medical exercise therapy

! +++
R 2 times a week, up to 4 weeks
PhysApps, ThE, MET

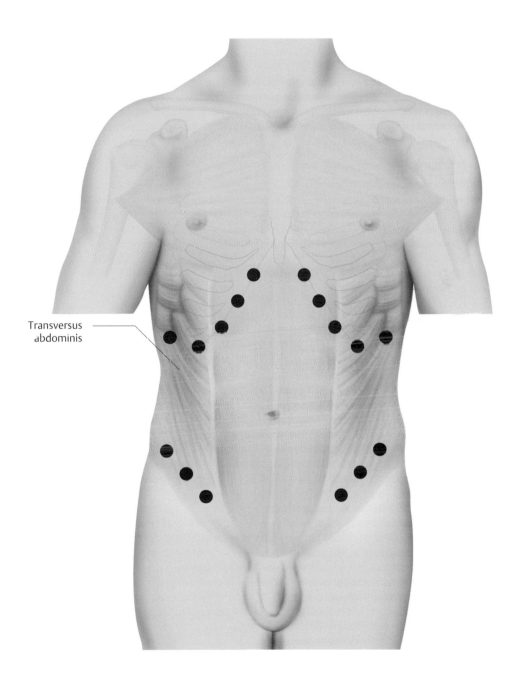

Transversus
abdominis

● Primarily Indicated injection points

Area of pain distribution

■ Therapy through the Skin

Disorders of the Stomach and the Duodenum

Indications

- Dysfunctions of the digestive tract
- Chronically recurring gastritis symptoms
- Irritations of the duodenum
- Acid reflux
- Pylorus spasms

Differential Diagnoses

- Malignant stomach diseases must be ruled out
- Ulcerations must be ruled out

Material

- Local anesthetic: 3 mL
- Needle: 0.4 × 20 mm

Technique

- Starting at the xiphoid process, injections are performed every 3 cm along the left costal arch up to the mamillary line. An intracutaneous quaddle containing 1 mL of a local anesthetic is set. The needle is then advanced superiorly until bone contact is made. Then, 0.3–0.5 mL of a local anesthetic is injected epiperiosteally. This procedure is repeated every 3 cm.
- Another injection is performed 2 cm inferior to the xiphoid process on the median line. After an intracutaneous quaddle has been set, the needle is advanced 0.5 cm and 0.5 ml of local anesthetic is injected. This procedure is repeated 2 cm inferior and again between the most lateral site of the subcostal injections and the most inferior site along the median line.

Risks

- If the needle is advanced excessively, abdominal organs may be injured.

Concomitant Therapies

- Regulation therapy, depending on the primary disorder
- Dietary therapy
- Behavior therapy
- Clarification through an internist or general practitioner

! ++
R 1–2 times a week, up to 6 weeks
Psy, Int, Gen, Nut

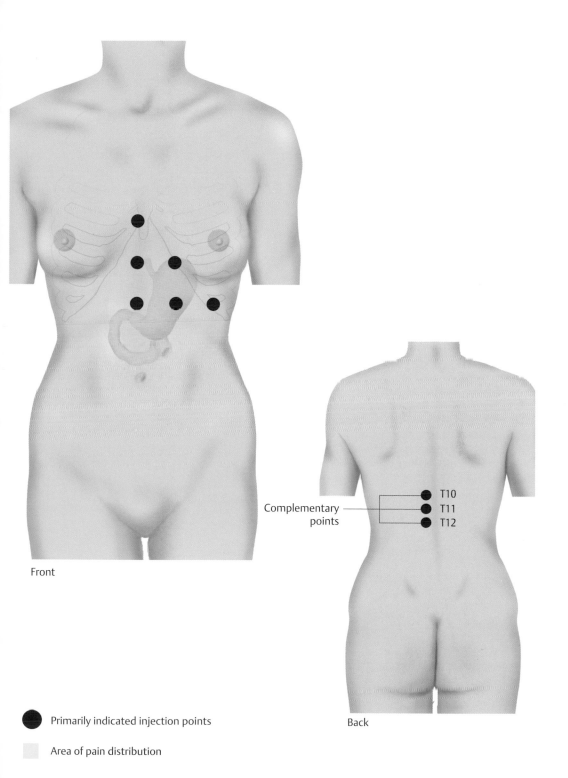

Complementary points — T10
T11
T12

Front

Back

● Primarily indicated injection points

Area of pain distribution

Pancreatic Pain Syndrome

Indications

- Chronically radiating pain originating in the pancreas
- Digestive disorders

Differential Diagnoses

- Obstructed outward flow from the major duodenal papilla. Caution: malignancies!
- Retroperitoneal affections, for example, migrating abscesses

Material

- Local anesthetic: 7 mL
- Needle: 0.6 × 30 mm

Technique

- Two lines are drawn 3 cm apart. They begin in the area of the paramedian line of the back at the level of the 11th/12th rib and travel beltlike slightly inferiorly, until they reach the navel. Along these lines, the needle is inserted vertically every 5 cm. First, an intracutaneous quaddle containing 0.1–0.2 mL of a local anesthetic is set. After the needle has been advanced 1 cm, 0.5 mL of a local anesthetic is injected.

Risks

- If the needle is advanced excessively, abdominal organs may be injured.
- Intensification of symptoms in inflammatory pancreatopathy

Concomitant Therapies

- Especially enzyme therapies, regulating dietary therapy
- Body wraps
- Clarification by an internist or general practitioner
- Surgical treatment in obstructed outward flow conditions, if applicable

---

! ++
R 2 times a week, up to 8 weeks
Med, PhysApps, Gen, Int, Nut

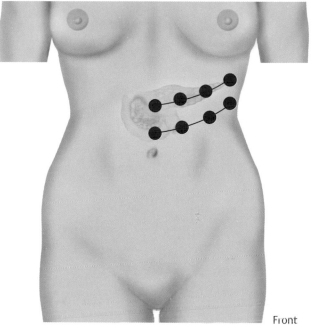

Front

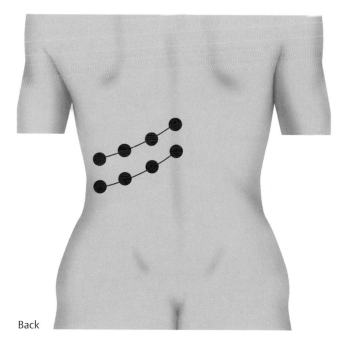

Back

● Primarily indicated injection points

  Area of pain distribution

Kidneys and Urinary Tract

Indications

- Adjuvant treatment in chronically recurring pyelonephritis, ureteral irritation, for example, after passing kidney stones
- Adjuvant treatment in recurring urinary tract infections

Material

- Local anesthetic: 5 mL
- Needle: 0.6 × 60 mm

Technique

- The intercostal space between the 11th and the 12th rib is located. The first insertion site is found 3 cm paravertebrally. The second insertion site is found 5 cm superiorly. Both sites are located parallel to the spinous processes. Each time, the needle is inserted vertically 3 cm and 1 mL of a local anesthetic is injected.
- The palpating finger travels from the inferior site laterally until it reaches the 12th rib after approximately 5 cm. This is the third injection site. The needle points toward the 12th rib, is advanced 1 cm, and 1 mL of a local anesthetic is injected.
- The injection sites on the front of the body are located as follows: The 12th rib is located on the axillary line. From here, a line is drawn to the pubic symphysis. On this line, an intracutaneous quaddle containing 0.1–0.2 mL of a local anesthetic is set every 5 cm. After each quaddle has been set, the needle is advanced 1 cm and 0.5 mL of a local anesthetic is injected.

Risks

- On the anterior aspect of the body, 1 cm is the maximum distance for needle advancement.
- If the needle is advanced excessively, abdominal organs and the peritoneum may be injured.

Concomitant Therapies

- Warm and moist segmental compresses (T9–T12 and L1)
- Dietary therapy, including large quantities of fluids and diuretic teas
- Reflexotherapy of the feet
- Bach Flower Therapy (Rock Rose and Aspen)
- Acupuncture

! ++
R 2 times a week, up to 6 weeks
Med, PhysApps, Acu, Urol

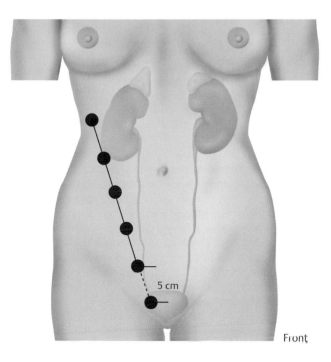

5 cm

Front

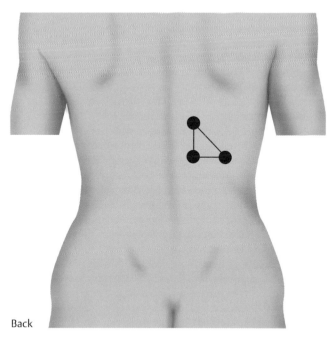

Back

● Primarily indicated injection points

▢ Area of pain distribution

Ovaries and Fallopian Tubes

Indications

- Recurring inflammation of the ovaries and fallopian tubes
- Pain syndromes during ovulation, painful ovarian cysts

Differential Diagnoses

- Tubal ectopic pregnancy
- Ovarian tumors

Material

- Local anesthetic: 2–3 mL
- Needle: 0.4 × 20 mm

Technique

- Treatment on the ovarian Y, the long side of which begins 2 finger widths superior to the anterior superior iliac spine and runs down to the pubic bone in a slight arch. This line is divided in three sections. The four injection sites are located at the ends of the line and the two division points. At each site, the needle is inserted vertically. A quaddle containing 0.1–0.2 mL of a local anesthetic is set, the needle is advanced 1 cm, and 0.5 mL of the injectable is administered.
- The additional site that completes the ovarian Y is located as follows: from the site second to the most superior one, a line is drawn toward the navel and from the most superior site a horizontal line is drawn medially; the injection site is found at the intersection of the two lines. Again, 0.1 mL of a local anesthetic is set intracutaneously, the needle is advanced 1 cm, and 0.5 mL of a local anesthetic is injected.

Risks

- If the needle is advanced excessively, abdominal organs may be injured.

Concomitant Therapies

- Moist heat application in the reflex segment; rising temperature hip baths; balm or mud treatment
- Reflexotherapy referring to the T10–L1 segment
- Phytotherapy using *Senecio ovatus* and evening primrose oil
- Transcutaneous electrical nerve stimulation, gynecological treatment

---

! ++
R 2 times a week, up to 8 weeks
PhysApps, TENS, MA, Med, Gyn

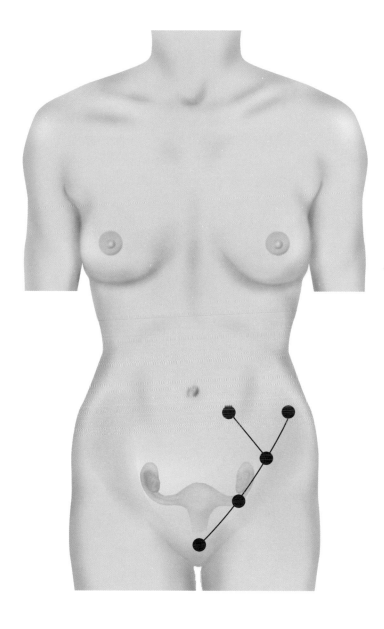

⬤ Primarily indicated injection points

▢ Area of pain distribution

Dysmenorrhea

Indications

- Menstrual disorders
- Chronic abdominal complaints
- Dysmenorrhea and irregular menstruation

Differential Diagnoses

- Bladder affections
- Pregnancy
- Genital neoplasms

Material

- Local anesthetic: 5 mL
- Needle: 0.6 × 60 mm

Technique

- Two quaddles are set intracutaneously superior to the symphysis, 1 cm to each side of the median line. They receive 0.1–0.2 mL of a local anesthetic. After the quaddles have been set, the needle is advanced 1 cm and 0.5 mL of the injectable is administered. This procedure is repeated at two sites 5 cm superior to the first two sites. The same procedure is repeated bilaterally, where a horizontal line that runs exactly in the middle of the four sites meets the ilium.
- It is recommended to add injections on the posterior aspect of the body, in the area of the rhombus of Michaelis. The first landmark is the posterior superior iliac spine; here, the needle is inserted and an intracutaneous quaddle is set. The needle is then advanced until bone contact is made and 0.5 mL of a local anesthetic is injected.
- On the median line, the inferior site is located slightly superior to the anal cleft. An injection of 0.5 mL of a local anesthetic at a depth of 1 cm at the level of the L4 spinous process completes the rhomboid shape formed by the injection sites.

Risks

- On the anterior aspect of the body, the bladder may be injured if the needle is advanced excessively; therefore, the depth of insertion must be observed.
- On the posterior aspect no risks are known.

Concomitant Therapies

- Intense exercises for the pelvic floor
- Assessment of the iliosacral joint using manual therapy as dysfunction of this joint frequently coexists
- Balm baths; rising temperature hip baths; local hay flower compresses on the anterior and the posterior aspect
- Abdominal shortwave therapy
- Gynecological treatment

! ++
R 3–4 times a week during the acute stage
ThE, MET, MM, Med, PhysApps, Gyn

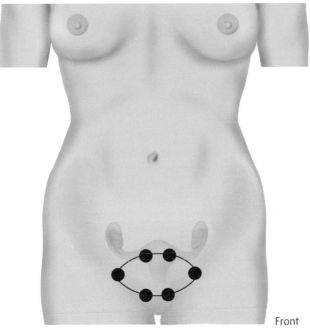

Front

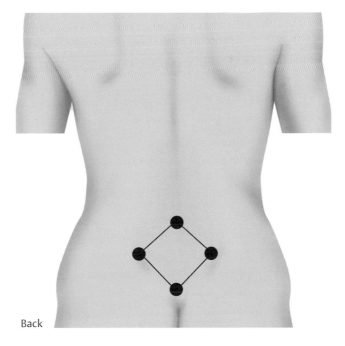

Back

● Primarily indicated injection points

  Area of pain distribution

Liver and Gallbladder Pain

Indications

- Dyskinesias of the bile ducts
- Hemopathy, right-sided functional complaints of the upper abdomen
- Chronic eructations
- Meteorism

Material

- Local anesthetic: 5 mL
- Needle: 0.6 × 60 mm

Technique

- Starting at the xiphoid process, along the right costal arch injections are performed in two rows, with the injection sites 3 cm apart. Each row comprises six injection sites. At each site, a quaddle of 0.1 mL is set, followed by the administration of 0.5 mL of a local anesthetic at a depth of 1 cm.
- Two finger widths paravertebrally, on the posterior aspect of the body, bilateral, two injections are performed at the level of T7/T8. The needle is inserted and immediately advanced 3 cm, at which point 1 mL of a local anesthetic is administered.

Concomitant Therapies

- Warm and moist segmental compresses
- Paravertebral and upper abdominal cupping
- Dietary therapy and therapeutic fasting
- Enzymatic treatment
- Drinking cures with sulfur water
- In spasms of the gallbladder, acupuncture at LU-2 and LU-3, GB-14, GB-37, and GB-38
- Periost massage along the right costal arch
- Internal medicine therapy, if applicable

! ++
R during the acute stage daily, up to 3 weeks
PhysApps, Nut, Med, Acu, FMA, Int

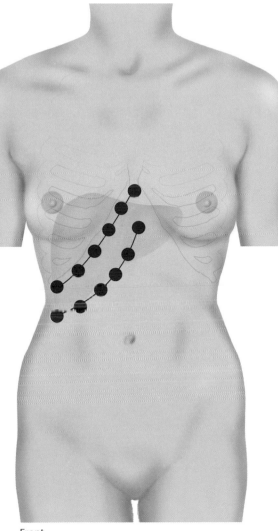

Front

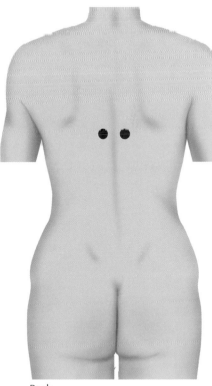

Back

Primarily indicated injection points

Area of pain distribution

6 Lumbar Spine and Pelvis

■ Complex Pain

Lumbago

Indications

- Pain conditions in lumbago and coxalgia
- Irritation of the gluteus maximus and the long back extensors
- Affections of the superior iliolumbar ligaments
- Tightening of the paravertebral muscles, as well as pseudoradicular symptoms

Differential Diagnoses

- Blockage of the sacroiliac joint and the L5 facet
- Inflammation of the sacroiliac joint
- Radicular symptoms in herniated vertebral disks
- Radiating complaints originating in disorders of the ureter and the bladder
- Referred pain originating in segmental processes (head zone T 11)
- Tumors in the lower abdomen
- Instability at the lumbosacral transition

Material

- Local anesthetic: 5–10 mL
- Needle: 0.8 × 80 mm

Technique

- The superior pelvic crest is palpated 2–3 finger widths paraspinally, at the level of the fifth lumbar vertebral body. The needle is inserted vertically until bone contact is made (transverse process of L5). A local anesthetic (2 mL) is injected. The needle is then retracted 1–2 cm and advanced toward the pelvic crest until bone contact is made. Here, the needle is retracted 2–3 mm and 2–3 mL of a local anesthetic is injected. The needle is inserted again, 2–3 finger widths inferior to the first injection site. The procedure of the first injection is repeated. This results in an almost isosceles triangle being formed.
- Complementary injections may be performed 1 finger width paraspinally next to L4/L5, L5/S1, and S1/S2, comprising a subcutaneous quaddle and an injection close to the bone. Equilateral injection at the greater trochanter is recommended if muscles connecting the pelvis and the greater trochanter are involved.

Risks

- Bone contact safeguards unintentional excessive advancement of the needle. If the needle is advanced too far centrally and drops after initial resistance, aspiration has to rule out unintentional administration near the spinal cord (liquor!).
- Direct infiltration between bone and periosteum should be avoided owing to its extreme painfulness.

Concomitant Therapies

- Dysfunctions of the sacroiliac joint are nearly always present; therefore, mobilization or manipulations of the sacroiliac joint are recommended.
- Relaxation techniques and muscular balancing by stretching the quadratus lumborum and muscles connecting the pelvis and the greater trochanter have been proven useful. The patient can repeat the exercises at home.
- Medical exercise therapy and physical therapy to relax the musculature.

! +++
R 2–3 times a week, up to 8 weeks
MM, ThE, MET, PhysApps, Chiro

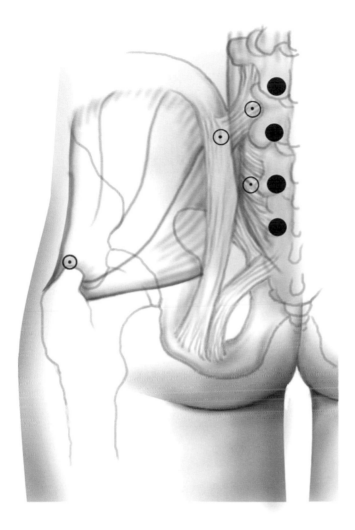

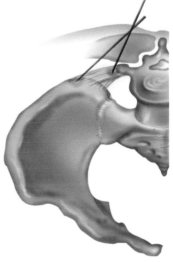

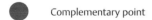

Complementary point

Points of deep injection

Area of pain distribution

Piriformis Syndrome

Indications

- Frequently, pseudoradicular symptoms in terms of sciatica. Patients complain about pain on the side of the hip when they are lying down at night.
- Tendinopathy of the greater trochanter
- Concomitant treatment of sacroiliac joint dysfunctions

Differential Diagnoses

- Sciatic irritations
- Affections of the gluteus medius

Material

- Local anesthetic: 5 mL
- Needle: 0.8 × 80 mm

Technique

- The greater trochanter is located. At its tip and 2 cm apart, along its posterior edge, the needle is inserted vertically until bone contact is made. After the needle has been retracted 1–2 mm, 1 mL of a local anesthetic is injected at each site.
- At the center, between the greater trochanter and the sacroiliac joint, the trigger point of the piriformis can be found. This is usually a painful area, including a rough palpable myogelosis. The needle is inserted 4 cm and 2 mL of the injectable is administered.

Risks

- If the needle is advanced excessively, the sciatic nerve may be anesthetized; therefore, the needle must be retracted if radiating, flashlike sensations are reported.

Concomitant Therapies

- Manual therapy in functional disorders of the sacroiliac joint
- Physical therapy in terms of stretching of the piriformis, including postisometric relaxation and instructions for self-mobilization. Differences in the length of the legs must be observed!

! +++
R 3 times a week, up to 6 weeks
MM, MA, ThE, Orthotech

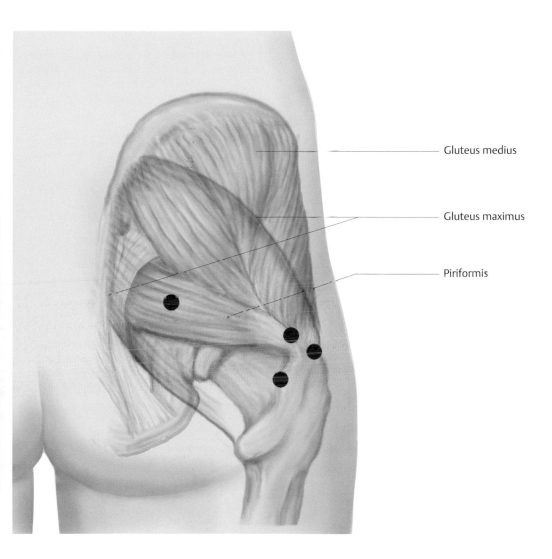

Gluteus medius

Gluteus maximus

Piriformis

● Primarily indicated injection points

  Area of pain distribution

Periarthritis Coxae

Indications

- Diffuse pain in the hip joint, pain accompanying hip arthrosis
- Adjuvant treatment in necrosis of the femoral head
- Treatment after placement of a total hip endo-prosthesis
- Treatment after femoral neck fracture

Differential Diagnoses

- Coxitis
- Metastases in older patients

Material

- Local anesthetic: 5 mL
- Needle: 0.8 × 80 mm

Technique

- Preferably with the patient in the lateral position, the tip of the greater trochanter is located. The needle is inserted vertically until bone contact is made. After the needle has been retracted slightly, 0.5 mL of a local anesthetic is injected. This procedure is repeated at the anterior and the posterior edge of the greater trochanter.
- With the patient in the supine position, with the legs slightly adducted, the pelvic adductor and gracilis attachment are located (from an abducted position, pressing the legs together against resistance). The needle is inserted until bone contact is made and 0.5 mL of a local anesthetic is injected 3–4 times in a semicircular pattern.
- An additional injection is located slightly distally to the intersection of a vertical line through the anterior superior iliac spine and a horizontal line coming from the tip of the greater trochanter. Another way to locate the insertion site is to move 2 cm lateral of the palpable pulse of the femoral artery, and 2 cm inferior of the inguinal ligament. The needle is inserted 3 cm and 2 mL of a local anesthetic is injected.

Risks

- Injection into the femoral artery; therefore, the easily palpable pulse must be observed. This risk can be avoided by aspiration prior to every injection.
- Anesthesia of the femoral nerve. The needle is retracted if flashlike sensations in the thigh are reported. The insertion is repeated further laterally.

Concomitant Therapy

- Physical therapy including sling exercise therapy on a table
- Thermal-bath-exercise therapy, hip traction treatment
- Orthopedic technical supply, for example, with heel cushions
- Medical exercise therapy
- Iontophoresis
- Transcutaneous electrical nerve stimulation (TENS)
- Thigh affusion according to Kneipp

! ++
R 1–2 times a week, up to 12 weeks
ThE, Orthotech, TENS, PhysApps, MET

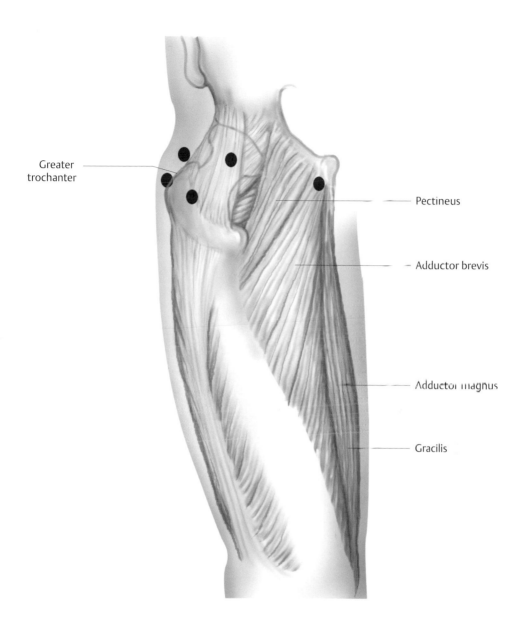

Greater trochanter

Pectineus

Adductor brevis

Adductor magnus

Gracilis

● Primarily indicated injection points

Area of pain distribution

■ Therapy through Muscles, Tendons, and Ligaments

Adductors

Indications

- Insertion tendinopathy of the adductor muscles near the pelvis

Differential Diagnoses

- Obturator irritation
- Inguinal and femoral hernia

Material

- Local anesthetic: 2 mL
- Needle: 0.6 × 60 mm

Technique

- The adductor group masses in a fan-shaped pattern near the pubic symphysis. While the legs are slightly abducted, the adductor group is palpated up to the pelvic edge, where the needle is inserted. The needle points toward the bone and is advanced until bone contact is made. In a fan-shaped pattern, 0.5 mL of a local anesthetic is injected 3–4 times close to the periosteum.
- If applicable, additional injection in the area of the medial attachment of the gracilis (see knee joint pain syndrome, p. 132)

Risks

- If the injectable is administered too close to the hip joint, the obturator nerve may be anesthetized and the obturator artery injured. This risk can be safely avoided by making bone contact with the needle prior to injection.

Concomitant Therapy

- Assessment of pelvic obliquity and sacroiliac joint dysfunction; if applicable, assessment of improper strain during athletic activities, including warm-up and cool-down phases
- In muscular imbalances, medical exercise therapy
- Cryotherapy and transverse friction massage
- Ultrasound therapy

! +++
R 2–3 times a week, up to 6 weeks
FMA, ThE, PhysApps, MET

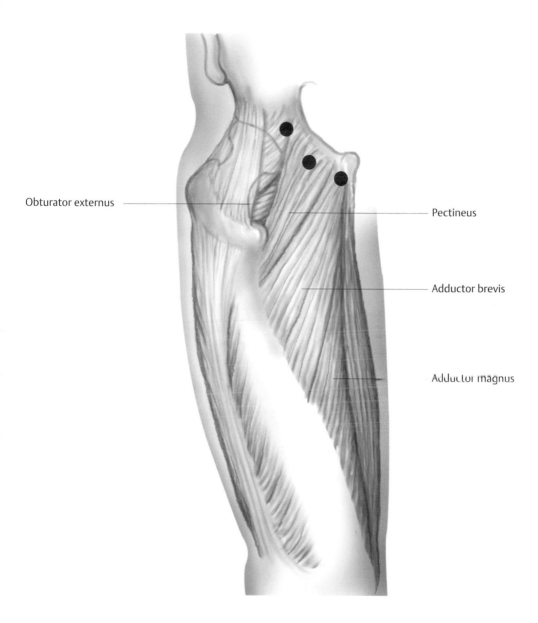

Obturator externus

Pectineus

Adductor brevis

Adductor magnus

● Primarily indicated injection points

  Area of pain distribution

Painful Long Back Extensors
(Longissimus, Iliocostalis)

Indications

- Thoracic and lumbar pain syndromes, especially in patients with a seated work position
- Chronic lumbago without radiating into the legs
- Painful spinous process
- Adjuvant treatment in the thoracic area for respiratory disorders
- Adjuvant treatment in the lumbar area for retroperitoneal disorders

Material

- Local anesthetic: 5–10 mL
- Needle: 0.6 × 60 mm

Technique

- In the thoracic area, injections are performed in one row, 1 finger width lateral to the spinous processes. The injection sites of this row are located 3 cm apart. The needle is inserted vertically 3 cm and 0.5 mL of a local anesthetic is injected.
- A second row of injections is shifted 4 cm inferior and 2 cm lateral to the first row. The procedure is repeated, but the depth of insertion here is only 1 cm!
- In the lumbar area, the first row of injections is 1 cm paravertebrally at the level of the palpable spinous processes. The second row of injections is 5 cm laterally and 5 cm superiorly up to the costal attachment. The needle is inserted vertically, on the paravertebral row 3 cm, and on the lateral row 1 cm. With each injection, 0.5 mL of a local anesthetic is administered.

Risks

- None if the depth of insertion is observed.
- If the needle is advanced excessively on the lateral insertion rows, pleura or retroperitoneal injuries may occur.

Concomitant Therapies

- Warm peloid applications
- High-frequency diathermy
- Relaxing massage
- Partial baths, jet blitz according to Kneipp
- Acupuncture along the bladder channel
- Balancing of the musculature using physical therapy
- Assessment and correction of working positions through occupational medicine
- Back training

! +++
R 2–3 times a week, up to 8 weeks
PhysApps, Acu, MET, ThE, Orthotech

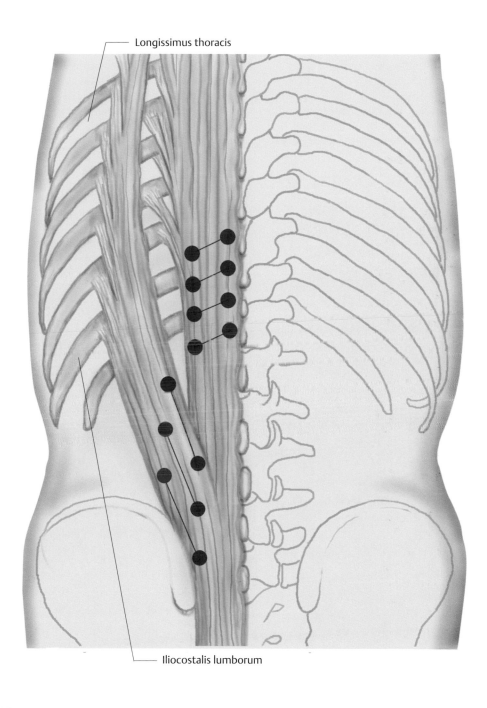

Longissimus thoracis

Iliocostalis lumborum

● Primarily indicated injection points

Area of pain distribution

■ Therapy through Nerves

Obturator Nerve

Indications

- Radiating hip pain, hip arthrosis, necrosis of the femoral head, phantom pain
- Persisting pain after surgical treatment of inguinal and femoral hernia

Material

- Local anesthetic: 7 mL
- Needle: 0.7 × 70 mm

Technique

- The patient is in the supine position with the legs slightly abducted. The insertion site is located 1.5 cm lateral and inferior to the palpable pubic tubercle. The needle is directed laterally and slightly superiorly toward the obturator canal. The needle is advanced up to the superior pubic ramus. After bone contact has been made, the needle feels its way inferiorly, until the obturator canal is reached. After prior aspiration, 5–7 mL of a local anesthetic is injected.

Risks

- Unintentional administration into the femoral artery and vein, the great saphenous vein, or the medial circumflex femoral artery. This risk can be safely avoided through aspiration prior to injection.

Concomitant Therapies

- Stretching of the pectineus and the obturator externus (postisometric relaxation) using physical therapy
- In chronic neuralgia, vitamin B supplements; if applicable, anti-inflammatories with systemic effect

> ! +++
> R 3 times a week, up to 4 weeks
> ThE, PIR, Med

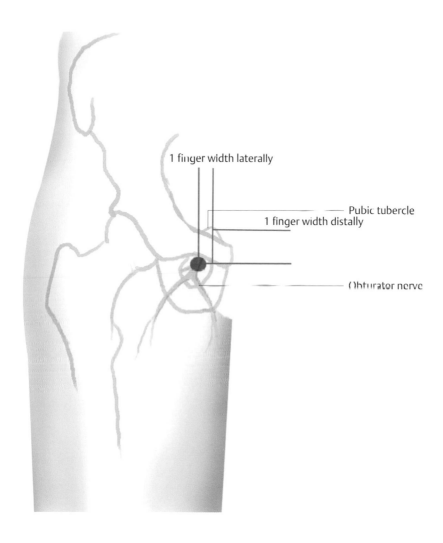

1 finger width laterally

Pubic tubercle

1 finger width distally

Obturator nerve

 Primarily indicated injection points

Area of pain distribution

Lateral Femoral Cutaneous Nerve

Indications

- Meralgia paresthetica nocturna, chronic irritation of the inguinal ligament
- Adjuvant treatment in persisting complaints after surgical treatment of inguinal and femoral hernia

Material

- Local anesthetic: 5 mL
- Needle: 0.6 × 60 mm

Technique

- The patient is in the supine position. The anterior superior iliac spine is palpated. The injection site is located 2 cm medially and 2 cm inferior to it. The needle is inserted vertically and advanced until contact with the fascia of musculus quadriceps femoris is made.
- After contact with the fascia has been made, a deposit is placed beneath it.

Risks

- None

Concomitant Therapies

- Vitamin B supplements
- Local TENS therapy
- Acupuncture on the liver channel (LV-10, LV-12) and on the stomach channel (ST-30, ST-31)
- Local cantharis plaster
- Relaxation of the hip flexors
- Surgical treatment, if persistent

! +++
R 2–3 times a week, up to 4 weeks; if applicable, one of the injections may contain low-dose corticosteroid
Med, PhysApps, Acu, ThE

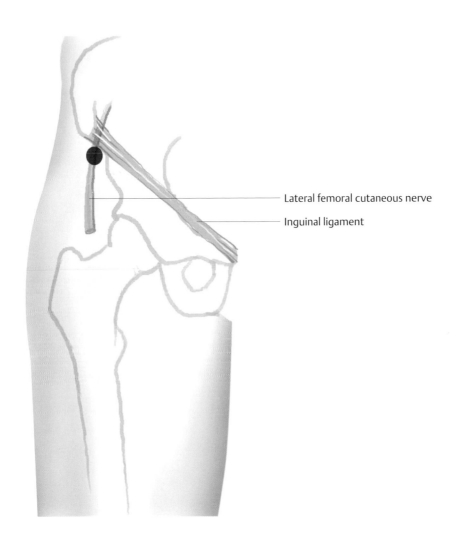

Lateral femoral cutaneous nerve

Inguinal ligament

● Primarily indicated injection points

Area of pain distribution

■ Therapy through Joints

Lumbar Vertebral Joints

Indications

- Facet arthrosis
- Lumbar pain intensified through increased lor-
  dosis

Differential Diagnoses

- Radicular symptoms
- Interspinous neoarthrosis

Material

- Local anesthetic: 5 mL at each level
- Needle: 0.9 × 90 mm

Technique

- The patient is in the flexed seated position or in
  the prone position with a pillow under the
  abdomen.
- Palpation and marking of the following points:
  spinous processes L5, L4, and L3; 2 cm lateral
  on a horizontal line between spinous processes
  L5, L4, and L3; 2 cm paralumbar vertically
  6–9 cm deep until bone contact is made.
- Injection of 2 mL of a local anesthetic at each
  side and for each joint.

Risks

- Peridural injection may occur if the needle is
  inserted too close to the median line. If the needle is inserted too far laterally, the corresponding spinal nerve may be anesthetized. It is
  imperative for the needle to make contact with
  bone prior to injection of the local anesthetic.

Concomitant Therapies

- Relaxation of the multifidus
- Inflecting lumbar orthosis
- Temporary resting position, supine with hips
  and knees flexed 90°, lower legs supported
- Strengthening of the anterior muscle chain

! +++
R 1–2 times a week
Orthothech, Acu, Chiro, PhysApps

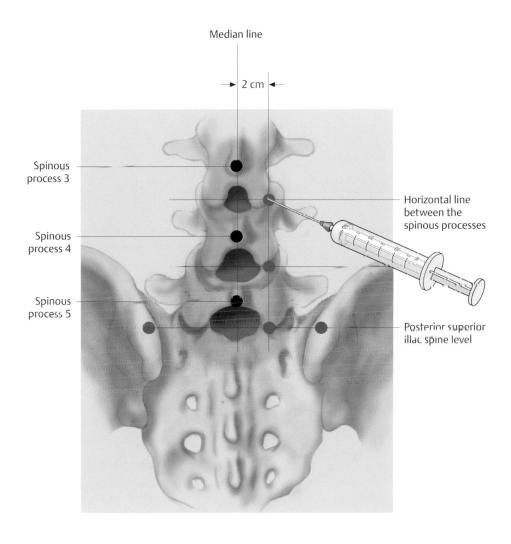

Median line

2 cm

Spinous
process 3

Spinous
process 4

Spinous
process 5

Horizontal line
between the
spinous processes

Posterior superior
iliac spine level

● Primarily indicated injection points

Area of pain distribution

7 Lower Extremities

■ Complex Pain

Patellofemoral Pain Syndrome (Runner's Knee)

Indications

- Irritation of the patellar ligament and the distal area of musculus quadriceps femoris
- Patellar chondropathy and arthrosis of the knee joint
- Pes anserinus tendinosis
- Patellar tendinitis (jumper's knee)
- Irritation of the infrapatellar nerve

Differential Diagnoses

- Inflammation of the knee joint (gonarthritis)
- Referred pain in disorders of the rectus femoris
- Referred pain in shortening of the vastus lateralis
- Radiating pain in inflammatory changes of the sural nerve and radicular symptoms in the L4 segment

Material

- Local anesthetic: 3–5 mL
- Needle: 0.4 × 40 mm

Technique

- The needle is inserted on the median line, inferior to the easily palpable patellar tip and is advanced approximately 1–1.5 cm. Following aspiration (to avoid intra-articular injection), 1–1.5 mL of a local anesthetic is injected.
- The next injections are performed in the pain area, approximately 1 finger width next to the midline, on the medial aspect of the knee. 1–1.5 mL of a local anesthetic is injected at points 1–1.5 cm apart across the joint, with the patient's knee extended. The needle is inserted only 0.5–1 cm. Aspiration is vital to avoid intra-articular injection.
- In addition, superior to the patella, medially and laterally to the attachment site of the rectus femoris, 1 mL of a local anesthetic is injected. The borders of the muscle can be easily palpated by having the patient lift the extended leg.

Risks

- Unintentional intra-articular injection occurs very easily. Superficial injection suffices at this location; therefore, the insertion depth of 0.50–1 cm must not be exceeded and prior aspiration is required.

Concomitant Therapies

- Depending on the underlying disorder, physical strain must be adjusted through corrections to the soles of shoes (internal and external sole lift) and adjustments regarding the foot statics or leg length. Frequently, especially in younger patients, considerable imbalance of the vastus medialis and the vastus lateralis can be seen. This requires adjuvant strengthening exercises for the vastus medialis. If the tibiofibular joint is affected, joint mobilization through manual therapy is recommended.
- In persistent irritations and positive McMurray test result or Cooper sign, the joint should be assessed using arthroscopy or MRI. Osteochondritis dissecans and osteochondral necrosis may be ruled out using radiologic assessment.
- In acute pain, temporary respite from athletic activities is recommended.
- In knee pain without organic correlation but with headache, a combination of acupuncture points ST-36, close to the knee, and ST-6, ST-8, and LI-4 has been successful.
- Additional injection of 0.5 mL of a local anesthetic in the area of GB-34 and GB-40, *yuan* source point, is helpful. Always inquire about functional disorders of the lumbar spine in combination with headache.

> ! ++
> R 1–2 times a week, up to 12 weeks
> Orhtotech, ThE, MET, MM, Acu

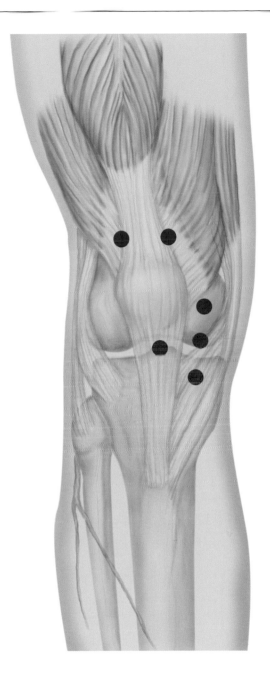

● Primarily indicated injection points

● Complementary point

Area of pain distribution

Gracilis and Pes Anserinus Pain Syndromes

Indications

- Median knee attachment tendinosis
- Overstrain syndrome of the knee joint capsule
- Adjuvant treatment in median gonarthritis

Material

- Local anesthetic: 3 mL
- Needle: 0.4 × 40 mm

Technique

- With the patient's knee in extension, a strong tapering muscular bulge at the medial joint line can be palpated. If it is palpated distally, its attachment at the tibial head is located. Here, the needle is inserted pointing superiorly and the attachment area is flooded with a local anesthetic in a fan-shaped pattern.
- On a vertical cranial line that initially deviates slightly posteriorly, two to three additional intracutaneous quaddles are set 2 cm apart. Each quaddle receives 0.2 mL of the injectable.

Risks

- Anesthesia of the saphenous nerve and its infra-patellar branch
- Intra-articular injection
- Intra-articular injection can be safely avoided if the needle is inserted as indicated, cranially at a shallow angle. If the saphenous nerve is temporarily anesthetized, the patient must be informed about the temporary characteristics.

Concomitant Therapies

- Iontophoretic treatment, local cryogenic friction massage
- Relaxation of the sartorius, semitendinosus, and gracilis using physical therapy
- Anti-inflammatory occlusive bandage
- Alternating knee affusion according to Kneipp

! +++
R 3 times a week, up to 6 weeks
PhysApps, FMA, ThE, MET

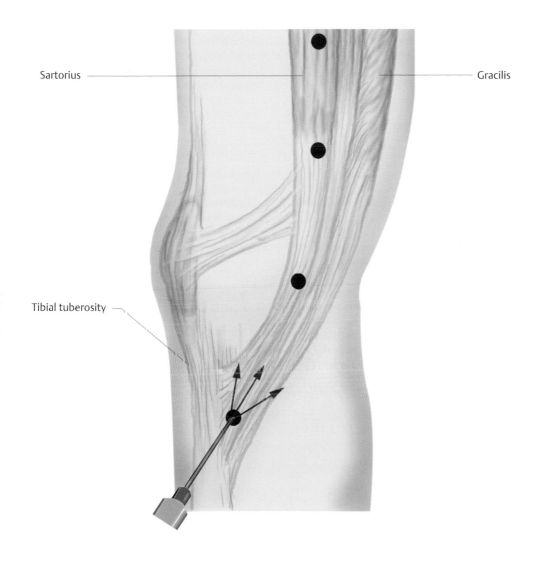

Sartorius

Gracilis

Tibial tuberosity

● Primarily indicated injection points

Area of pain distribution

■ Therapy through Muscles, Tendons, and Ligaments

Biceps Femoris

Indications

- Painful lateral edge of the knee joint, painful fibular head
- Myotenositis of the biceps femoris

Differential Diagnoses

- Lesion of the lateral meniscus
- Irritation of the infrapatellar nerve
- Maisonneuve fracture

Material

- Local anesthetic: 2 mL
- Needle: 0.4 × 40 mm

Technique

- The fibular is easily located through palpation. The needle is inserted 1 cm superior, pointing toward the fibular head.
- After bone contact has been made, the injectable is administered as the needle is retracted.

Risks

- Anesthesia of the peroneus nerve. The nerve reaches the fibular head from posteriorly, and spirals around it in a superior direction. Anesthesia of the peroneus nerve can be safely avoided if the needle makes bone contact prior to injection.

Concomitant Therapies

- Mobilization of the tibiofibular joint using manual therapy
- Friction massage
- Ultrasound applications
- Cryotherapy
- Acupuncture (ST-36, ST-35)

! ++
R 2 times a week, up to 4 weeks
MM, FMA, PhysApps, Acu

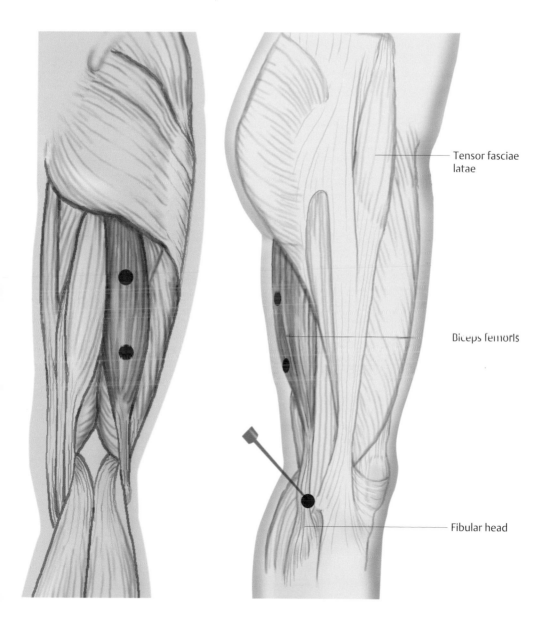

Tensor fasciae latae

Biceps femoris

Fibular head

● Primarily indicated injection points

  Area of pain distribution

Quadriceps Femoris

Indications

- Pain appears especially near the knee joint superior to the patella and in terms of lower patellar pole syndromes.
- Adjuvant treatment in patellar chondropathy and retropatellar arthrosis

Differential Diagnoses

- Free joint body
- Prepatellar bursitis
- Gonarthrosis, gonarthritis

Material

- Local anesthetic: 3 mL
- Needle: 0.4 × 44 mm

Technique

- The superior edge of the patella is palpated and three or four injections are performed superior to the palpable bony edge. First an intracutaneous quaddle is set, the needle is then advanced 0.5 cm, and 0.3 mL of a local anesthetic is injected at each site.
- In the area of the inferior patellar pole, the procedure is repeated. The insertion is directed toward the bone. Below the bone, close to the patellar periosteum, 0.5 mL of a local anesthetic is injected. The depth of insertion is 0.5 cm.
- Finally, in the area of the palpable tibial tuberosity, a quaddle is set at its superior edge. The needle is then advanced until bone contact is made. After the needle has been retracted 1 mm, 0.5 mL of a local anesthetic is injected.

Risks

- Unintentional intra-articular injection; this can be avoided by observing the depth of insertion and making bone contact with the needle prior to injection.

Concomitant Therapies

- Traction mobilization of the patella
- In muscular imbalances, it is frequently necessary to strengthen the vastus medialis through exercises.
- Prescription of quadriceps support aids, for example, negative heel
- Priessnitz compress
- Medical exercise therapy

! +++
R 2 times a week, up to 8 weeks
MM, ThE, MET, Orthotech, PhysApps

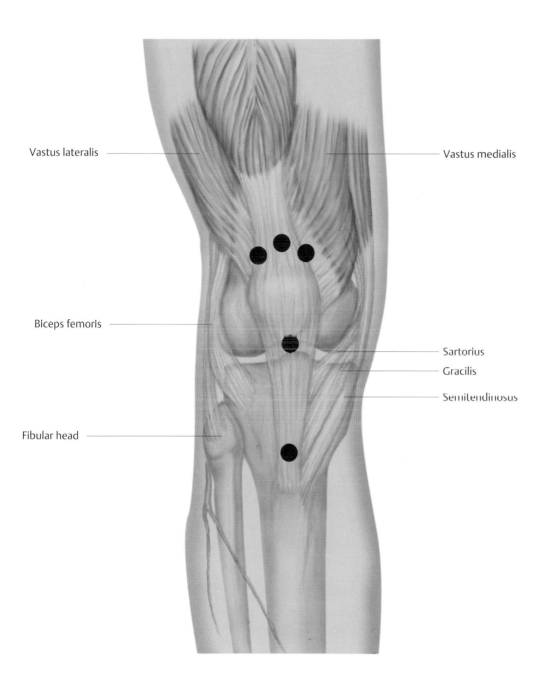

Vastus lateralis

Vastus medialis

Biceps femoris

Sartorius

Gracilis

Semitendinosus

Fibular head

Primarily indicated injection points

Area of pain distribution

Triceps Surae

Indications

- Calf pain, radiating into the Achilles tendon
- Adjuvant treatment in:
  - achillodynia
  - knee flexion contracture
  - contracted drop foot
  - calf cramps at night

Differential Diagnoses

- Venous insufficiency
- Deep vein thrombosis
- Compartment syndrome
- Peripheral arterial occlusion

Material

- Local anesthetic: 5 mL
- Needle: 0.5 × 50 mm

Technique

- The patient is in the pronated position and attempts plantar flexion of the foot against resistance. This requires tensing the gastrocnemius and the soleus. The superior border of the two gastrocnemius heads is located. The needle is inserted 2 cm and 0.5 mL of a local anesthetic is injected on each side.
- Five centimeters distally, on top of the muscle bellies, the needle is inserted 2 cm and 0.5 mL of a local anesthetic is injected bilaterally. The needle is then advanced another 2 cm and the injectable is administered again.
- The distal conjunction of the gastrocnemius heads is located. A notch on the median line indicates the precise injection site. The needle is inserted vertically 2 cm and 0.5 mL of a local anesthetic is injected.

Risks

- Injection into the small saphenous vein
- If the needle is advanced excessively, the tibial nerve may be anesthetized.

Concomitant Therapies

- Muscular relaxation using physical therapy
- Connective-tissue massage
- Traction mobilization of the knee joint and the ankle joint
- Supportive heel lift, if applicable
- Calf affusion according to Kneipp
- Priessnitz compress, cupping therapy

! ++
R 3 times a week, up to 6 weeks
ThE, MA, MM, Orthotech, PhysApps

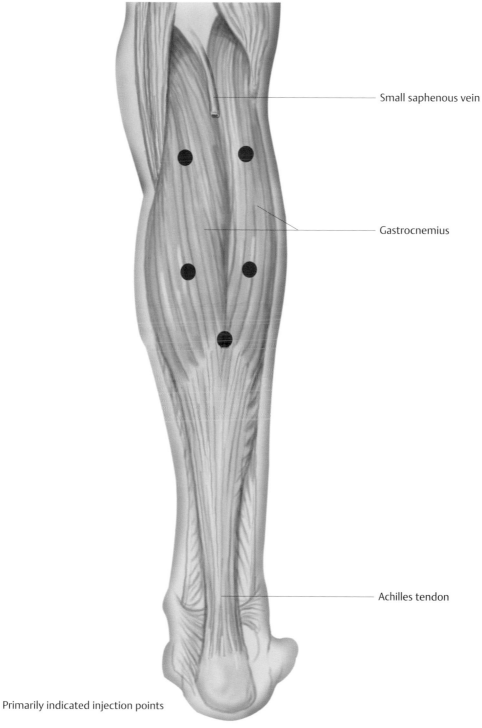

Small saphenous vein

Gastrocnemius

Achilles tendon

Primarily indicated injection points

Area of pain distribution

Peronei

Indications

- Pain in the area of the lateral lower leg
- Pain along the course of the tendon at the lateral malleolus
- Adjuvant treatment in:
  - genua vara (bow legs)
  - dysfunction of the upper and lower ankle joints
  - partial weakness after disk herniation at L4/L5

Differential Diagnoses

- Compartment syndrome
- Peripheral arterial occlusion

Material

- Local anesthetic: 3 mL
- Needle: 0.4 × 40 mm

Technique

- The patient is in the lateral position. The prominent fibular head is palpated. The first injection is performed directly inferior to the fibular head, at the transition onto the muscle attachment. The needle is inserted vertically until bone contact is made. The needle is then retracted 1 mm and 0.5 mL of a local anesthetic is injected.
- On a straight line down to the lateral malleolus, two additional injections are performed 4 cm apart. The needle is inserted vertically 1 cm and 0.5 mL of a local anesthetic is administered.
- The final injection is performed posterior to the lateral malleolus. Nearly parallel to the peroneal tendon, the needle is inserted caudally at a shallow angle into the tendon sheath. Then, 0.5 mL of a local anesthetic is injected.

Risks

- If the injectable is administered posterior to the fibular head, the peroneal nerve may be anesthetized and temporary weakness in dorsal flexion of the foot may result.
- No additional risks are known.

Concomitant Therapies

- Dynamic exercises for plantar flexion
- Subfibular friction massage
- Priessnitz compress
- Shoe adjustment through external heel lift to support the peroneus
- Physical application in terms of analgesic electrotherapy

! ++
R 2 times a week, up to 8 weeks
MET, ThE, FMA, Orthotech, PhysApps

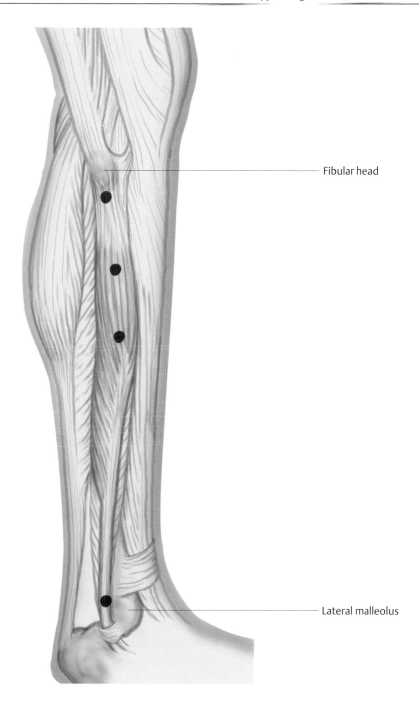

Fibular head

Lateral malleolus

● Primarily indicated injection points

  Area of pain distribution

Medial Collateral Ligament

Indications

- Conditions following:
  - distortion of the knee joint
  - partial rupture of the collateral ligament
  - surgical treatment of the collateral ligament
- Adjuvant radiating tendinosis

Differential Diagnoses

- Damage to the medial meniscus
- Osteochondritis dissecans
- Medial gonarthrosis

Material

- Local anesthetic: 2 mL
- Needle: 0.4 × 20 mm

Technique

- The palpable medial joint line is located. Along the course of the medial collateral ligament, 2 cm superior and inferior to the joint line, the needle is inserted vertically until bone contact is made.
- The needle is then retracted 1 mm and 0.5 mL of a local anesthetic is injected at the proximal and the distal attachment site.

Risks

- None

Concomitant Therapies

- Friction massage at the ligamental attachments, depending on the cause of the condition
- Local cryotherapy
- Measures to support the collateral ligament
- Transcutaneous electrical nerve stimulation (TENS)
- Acupuncture on the liver channel (LV-6, LV-7, LV-8, LV-9)
- Phonophoresis

! +++
R 3 times a week, up to 4 weeks
FMA, TENS, Orthotech, Acu, PhysApps

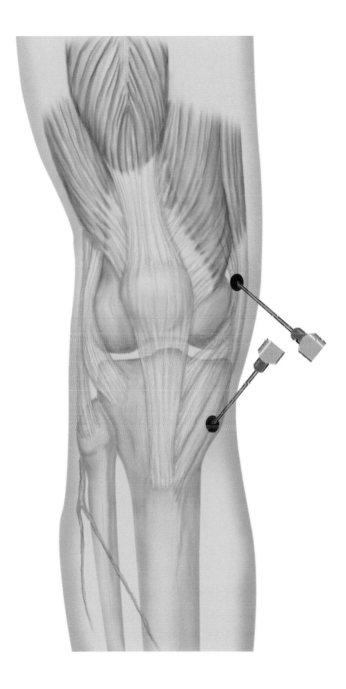

● Primarily indicated injection points

Area of pain distribution

Lateral Collateral Ligament

Indications

- Distortion of the lateral collateral ligament
- Partial rupture and conditions following surgical treatment
- Adjuvant tendinosis

Material

- Local anesthetic: 2 mL
- Needle: 0.4 × 20 mm

Technique

- The lateral joint line is palpated. With the knee slightly flexed, the ligament travels from the fibular head to the lateral epicondyle of the femur. The needle is inserted approximately 2 cm inferior to the palpable joint line, superior to the fibular head, until bone contact is made. The needle is then retracted 1 mm and 0.5 mL of a local anesthetic is injected.
- The procedure is repeated 2 cm superior to the joint line. The needle is inserted until bone contact is made, retracted 1 mm, and 0.5–1 mL of a local anesthetic is injected.

Risks

- If the needle is inserted too far posteriorly and advanced excessively in the area of the fibular head, the peroneus nerve may be anesthetized. This may result in temporary weakness in dorsal flexion of the foot. The insertion site must be precisely located.

Concomitant Therapies

- Friction massage according to Cyriax
- Local cryotherapy, reduction of strain on the lateral compartment
- Priessnitz compress
- Knee affusions, phonophoresis, shoe adjustment, correction of faulty foot statics

! +++
R 3 times a week, up to 4 weeks
FMA, PhysApps, Orthotech

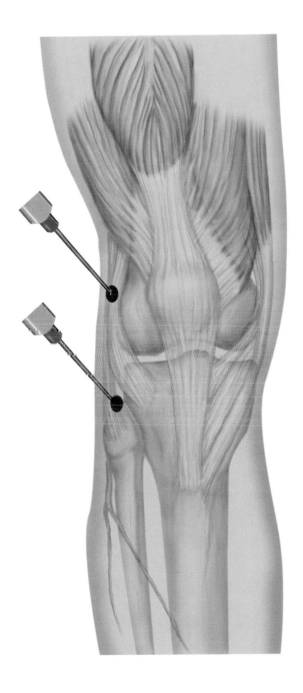

● Primarily indicated injection points

  Area of pain distribution

■ Therapy through Nerves

Infrapatellar Nerve

Indications

- Patellar chondropathy, pain syndromes of the tibial tubcrosity
- Adjuvant treatment in:
  - lesions of the medial meniscus
  - medial gonarthrosis

Material

- Local anesthetic: 3 mL
- Needle: 0.4 × 40 mm

Technique

- The infrapatellar branch of the saphenous nerve splits off the saphenous nerve directly superior to the tibial tuberosity and travels nearly horizontally to the knee. Insulated local anesthesia of the infrapatellar nerve requires the needle to be inserted caudally, anterior to the palpable end of the sartorius and inferior to the joint line.
- After the needle has been advanced 3 cm, the local anesthetic is continuously injected while the needle is being retracted.

Risks

- If the injection is performed too far posteriorly, the saphenous nerve may be anesthetized and unintentional injection into the great saphenous vein or artery may occur; therefore, aspiration is required prior to injection.

Concomitant Therapies

- Reduction of strain on the medial compartment through shoe adjustment (lateral heel lift), balancing the muscular command of the patella, reduction of strain on the patella
- Friction massage on the sartorius and gracilis
- Local application of essential oils

! +++
R 3 times a week, up to 4 weeks
Orthotech, ThE, MET, Med

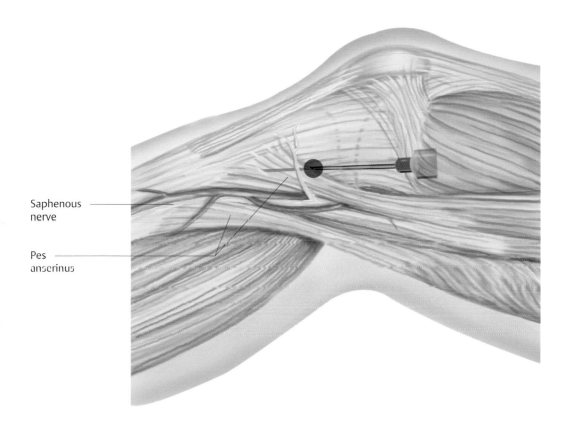

Saphenous
nerve

Pes
anserinus

● Primarily indicated injection points

Area of pain distribution

Tarsal Tunnel and Tibialis Posterior Compartment

Indication

- Tarsal tunnel syndrome
- Chronic ankle pain with decompensated pes valgus (splayfoot)
- Functional disorders and arthroses of the upper and lower ankle joints

Differential Diagnoses

- Arthritis of the upper ankle joint
- Achillodynia, traumatic injuries to the upper ankle joint
- Peripheral arterial occlusion

Material

- Local anesthetic: 3 mL
- Needle: 0.4 × 40 mm

Technique

- With the patient's foot externally rotated, the posterior tibial artery is palpated and landmarked. Insertion takes place between the medial malleolus and the easily palpable tibial artery. The needle is advanced 1.5 cm toward the foot until bone contact is made. After aspiration, 1.5 mL of the local anesthetic is injected.
- Owing to the anatomical variability of the nerve, the injection is repeated on the other side of the artery. The needle is inserted again directly next to the vessel and advanced 1.5 cm toward the foot. After negative aspiration, 1.5 mL of the local anesthetic is administered.

Risks

- Intravascular administration; therefore, aspiration is necessary prior to injection.

Concomitant Therapies

- Traction mobilization of the upper and lower ankle joints
- Iontophoresis
- Transcutaneous electrical nerve stimulation therapy over the tibial nerve
- Reduction of the strain on the foot through longitudinal arch support; exercising the intrinsic muscles
- Alternating hot and cold footbaths
- Sole baths

! +++
R 1–2 times a week, up to 4 weeks; if applicable, one of the injections may contain low-dose corticosteroid
MM, PhysApps, TENS, Orthotech, ThE

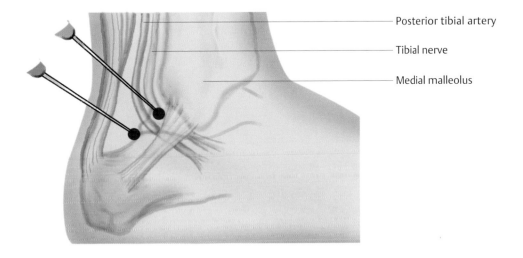

Posterior tibial artery

Tibial nerve

Medial malleolus

● Primarily indicated injection points

Area of pain distribution

Interdigital Nerve (Morton Neuroma)

Indications

- Interdigital pain, neuralgiform Morton symptoms
- Hallux valgus (bunion deformity), claw toe deformity accompanied by metatarsalgia
- Forefoot pain in faulty foot statics

Material

- Local anesthetic: 1 mL per interdigital space
- Needle: 0.4 × 20 mm

Technique

- On the dorsal aspect of the foot, the needle is inserted vertically 2 cm into the palpable interdigital space, and 1 mL of the injectable is administered per interdigital space.
- While the needle is being retracted, the local anesthetic is continuously injected to cover the interdigital nerves as well as the ligaments.

Risks

- None

Concomitant Therapies

- Mobilization of the metatarsophalangeal joints, mobilization of the transverse arch of the foot in splayfoot using manual therapy
- Reflexotherapy of the feet, compensation of faulty statics in splayfoot
- Transcutaneous electrical nerve stimulation, self-mobilization, for example, tennis ball, and supportive splayfoot bandage
- Surgical revision, if applicable

! +++
R 2 times a week, up to 6 weeks
MM, Orthotech, TENS

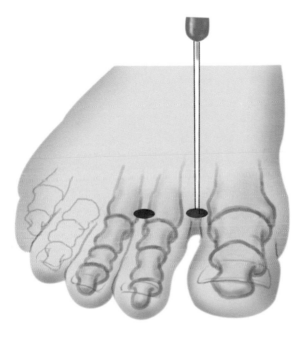

● Primarily indicated injection points

▢ Area of pain distribution

Calcaneus Pain

Indications

- Calcaneodynia
- Plantar fasciitis, plantar heel spur

Differential Diagnoses

- Tarsal tunnel syndrome
- Synostoses
- Referred radicular symptoms

Material

- Local anesthetic: 2 mL
- Needle: 0.4 × 40 mm

Technique

- The patient is in a supine position and the knee is flexed at a right angle. The anterior edge of the calcaneus is palpated. The needle is inserted toward the calcaneus, 1 cm medial to a longitudinal line that runs through the center of the foot.
- After bone contact has been made, the injectable is administered in a fan-shaped pattern at the periost.

Concomitant Therapies

- Temporary reduction of strain on the heel through soft foot bedding, accommodation of false foot statics
- Heel lift, iontophoresis, foot exercises, massage with small wooden sticks and cryotherapy, foot compress
- Extracorporeal shockwave lithotripsy

! +++
R 2–3 times a week, up to 12 weeks; if applicable, one of the injections may contain low-dose corticosteroid
Orthotech, PhysApps, ThE, ESWL

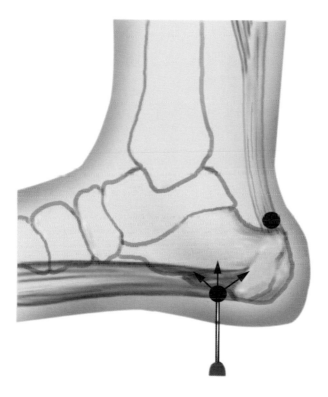

● Primarily indicated injection points

  Area of pain distribution

■ Therapy through the Skin

Knee Circle

Indications

- Patellar chondropathy
- Retropatellar arthrosis
- Dysfunction of the patellofemoral slide
- Conditions following surgical treatment

Differential Diagnoses

- Gonarthritis
- Prepatellar bursitis
- Free joint bodies

Material

- Local anesthetic: 3 mL
- Needle: 0.4 × 20 mm

Technique

- In a circle around the patella, intracutaneous quaddles each containing 1 mL of a local anesthetic are set. The distance between the patella and each injection site is 1 cm. The needle is then advanced until bone contact is made.
- After the needle has been retracted 1 mm, 0.2 mL of a local anesthetic is administered near the periosteum. This procedure is repeated all the way around the patella.

Risks

- None if the needle is inserted toward the patella.
- If the needle is inserted vertically, unintentional intra-articular injection into the recess may result; therefore, the tip of the needle must make contact with the patella.

Concomitant Therapies

- Mobilization of the patellofemoral slide using manual therapy
- Short-stretch bandages on the patella, if applicable
- Support in terms of orthopedic shoes
- Aquatic exercise therapy
- Thermal baths
- Strengthening of the vastus medialis using physical therapy
- Priessnitz compress

! ++
R 2 times a week, up to 12 weeks
MM, Orthotech, PhysApps, ThE, MET

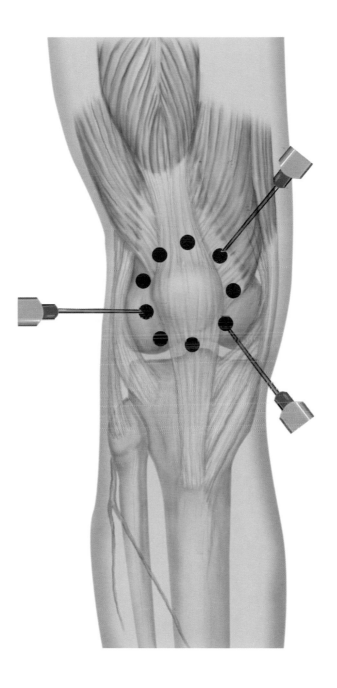

● Primarily indicated injection points

  Area of pain distribution

Medial Meniscus Pain

Indication

- Medial gonarthrosis
- Degeneration of the meniscus

Differential Diagnoses

- Tendinosis of the medial collateral ligament
- Tendinosis of the pes anserinus

Material

- Local anesthetic: 2 mL
- Needle: 0.4 × 20 mm

Technique

- Semicircularly, intracutaneous quaddles are set 2 cm apart along the palpable joint line of the knee, beginning parapatellarly and following the horizontal plane. Each quaddle contains 0.1 mL of a local anesthetic.
- After setting the quaddles, the needle is advanced 0.5 cm at each side and 0.2–0.3 mL of the local anesthetic is administered.

Risks

- If the needle is advanced excessively, unintentional intra-articular injection may occur; therefore, aspiration and the depth of insertion must be observed.

Concomitant Therapies

- Reduced strain on the medial compartment, for example, through an external heel lift or through traction mobilization of the joint
- Aquatic exercise therapies, local hyperemic treatment through iontophoresis
- Priessnitz compress

! ++
R 2 times a week, up to 12 weeks
Orthotech, MM, PhysApps

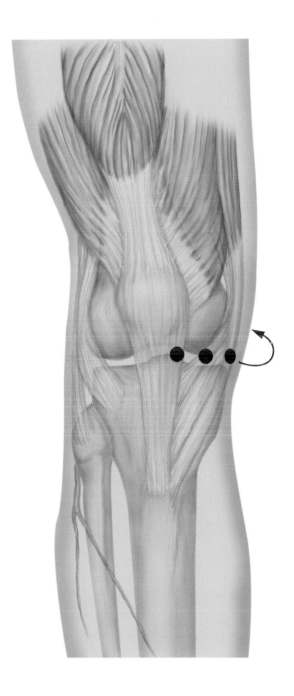

● Primarily indicated injection points

　 Area of pain distribution

Lateral Meniscus Pain

Indications

- Lateral meniscus pain syndromes
- Valgus gonarthrosis

Material

- Local anesthetic: 2–3 mL
- Needle: 0.4 × 20 mm

Technique

- Semicircularly, intracutaneous quaddles are set 2 cm apart along the palpable lateral joint line of the knee, beginning lateral to the patellar ligament and following the horizontal plane. Each quaddle contains 0.1 mL of a local anesthetic.
- After setting the quaddles, the needle is advanced 0.5 cm at each side and 0.2–0.3 mL of the local anesthetic is administered.

Risk

- If the needle is advanced excessively, unintentional intra-articular injection may occur; therefore, aspiration and the depth of insertion must be observed.

Concomitant Therapies

- Reduced strain on the lateral compartment, for example, through an internal heel lift
- Traction mobilization of the joint
- Aquatic exercise therapy
- Priessnitz compress
- Local anti-inflammatory and hyperemic applications, for example, iontophoresis

---

! +
R 2 times a week, up to 6 weeks
Orthotech, MM, PhysApps

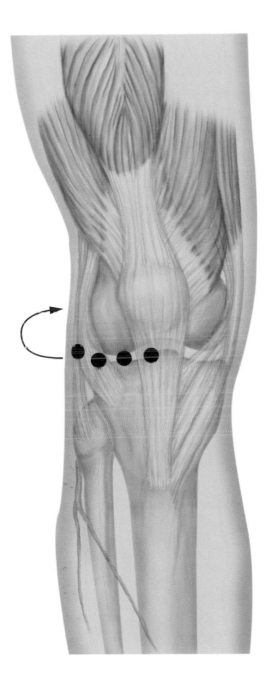

● Primarily indicated injection points

  Area of pain distribution

Pain along the Tibia

Indications

- Tibial periostoses
- Night cramps in the area of the anterior tibia

Differential Diagnoses

- Radicular symptoms in herniated disks
- Peripheral arterial occlusion

Material

- Local anesthetic: 3 mL
- Needle: 0.4 × 40 mm

Technique

- The anterior edge of the tibia is palpated. The first injection is performed directly inferior to the tibial tuberosity, lateral to the anterior edge of the tibia. The needle is inserted vertically and advanced until contact with the periosteum is made. After the needle has been retracted 1 mm, 0.5 mL of a local anesthetic is administered at the periosteum. Along the lateral aspect of the tibial edge, this procedure is repeated 4–5 times, at points 4 cm apart.

Risks

- None

Concomitant Therapies

- Frequently, false foot static is present in terms of flat foot (pes valgus) and overstrains the anterior tibialis. This requires supporting measures for the longitudinal arch.
- Lower leg affusions, friction massage in the area of the attachment of the anterior tibialis at the lateral aspect of the tibia.

! ++
R 2 times a week, up to 12 weeks
Orthotech, PhysApps, FMA

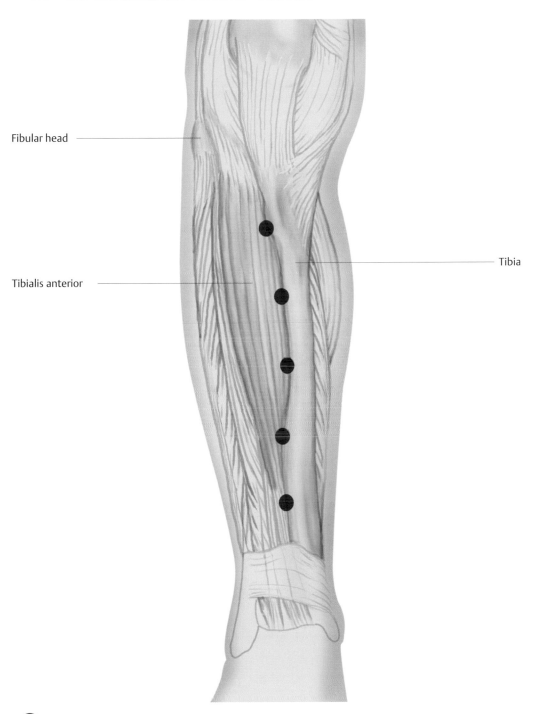

Fibular head

Tibialis anterior

Tibia

● Primarily indicated injection points

   Area of pain distribution

■ Therapy and Joint Injection

Hip Joint

Indications

- Arthritis, coxarthrosis

Differential Diagnoses

- Periarthritis coxae
- Tendinopathy of the trochanter
- Inguinal hernia

Material

- Local anesthetic: 6–7 mL
- Needle: 0.9 × 90 mm

Technique

- The patient is in a stable lateral position. The affected leg rests on top, is extended, and is positioned on a pillow in the neutral position.
- The greater trochanter is palpated approximately 10–15 cm caudal to the iliac crest. The cranial edge of the trochanter is palpated firmly and deeply, and the leg is passively abducted. When the leg is abducted, the palpating finger drops into a depression, which indicates the injection site.
- The needle is inserted vertically. During aspiration, the needle is advanced until bone contact is made. Immediately before the bone is reached, the joint capsule is penetrated and resistance ceases. The injection can be performed without applying force.

Risks

- The circumflex femoral artery may be injured; therefore, aspiration is vital. With intracapsular positioning of the needle tip, the injection can only be performed if considerable pressure is applied.

Concomitant Therapies

- Mobilization using manual therapy
- Hip traction treatments, systemic anti-inflammatory applications
- Support through forearm walking crutches, axial cushioning through buffer heels

---

! +++
R once a week
ThE, MM, Med, Orthotech

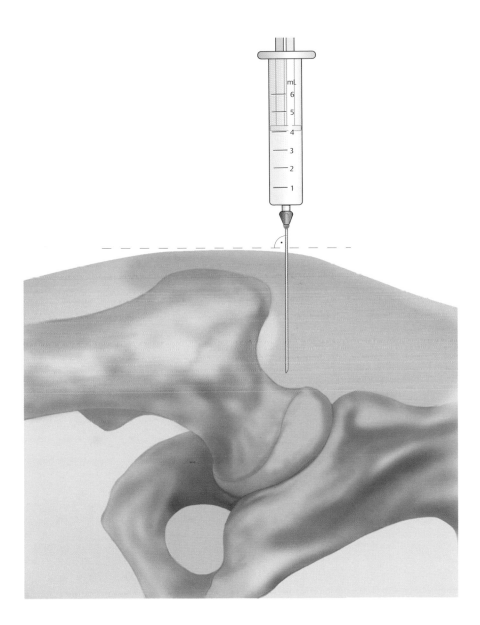

Knee Joint

Indications

- Arthritis
- Degenerative disorders
- Posttraumatic internal knee injuries

Material

- Local anesthetic: 10 mL
- Needle: 0.7 × 30 mm

Technique

- The patient sits with the knee in 90° flexion, and the leg hangs down without the foot resting on the floor. The medial and lateral joint line next to the knee joint is palpated and marked. The connecting line is the first auxiliary line. One centimeter lateral, the patellar tendon is then palpated (or 1 cm medial to the patellar tendon).
- The injection site is found at the intersection of the parapatellar line and the horizontal auxiliary line. The needle is inserted vertically and advanced 3 cm. Injection of a small amount of the local anesthetic indicates the precise intra-articular location of the needle tip.
- Moderate pressure must suffice to perform the injection. The tip of the needle is not positioned correctly if the patient reports sudden pain during the injection. This usually indicates the needle tip is located in the Hoffa fat pad. While applying gentle pressure onto the plunger, the physician moves the needle slightly back and forth, until the position for smooth injection is found.
- Never use force to administer the injectable.

Risks

- Injection into the Hoffa fat pad (resisted injection)

Concomitant Therapies

- Local cryotherapy
- Topical anti-inflammatory application
- Orthopedic support, axial cushioning through buffer heels
- Physical therapy
- TENS treatments
- NSAIDs with systemic effect

---

1 +++
R 1–2 times a week
Cryo, MM, Orthotech, TENS, PhysApps, Med

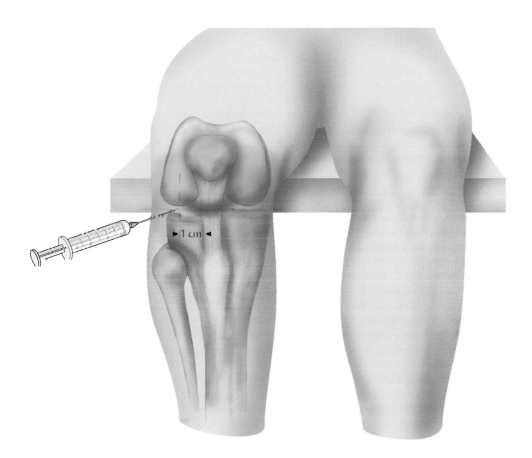

►1 cm◄

Upper Ankle Joint (Talocrural Articulation)

Indications

- Arthritis
- Arthrosis of the ankle joint
- Posttraumatic osteochondritis dissecans

Differential Diagnoses

- Tenosynovitis in the area of the extensor retinaculum
- Midfoot arthritis

Material

- Local anesthetic: 5 mL
- Needle: 0.6 × 30 mm

Technique

- The patient is in the supine position, the knee is in 45° flexion, and the foot is placed flat on the treatment surface. The medial and lateral malleolus is palpated. Palpation moves 1–1.5 cm cranially. During passive (!) alternating dorsal and plantar flexion, a depression can be palpated. Active movement of the foot prevents palpation of the joint line owing to the tightening of the extensor hallucis tendon.
- The horizontal joint line is marked. The tendon of the extensor hallucis is identified by raising the patient's big toe against resistance. The tendon of the anterior tibialis is easily located by lifting the medial side of the patient's foot. The injection site is located on the horizontal joint line between the two easily palpable tendons.
- The needle is not inserted vertically to the anterior tibial edge, but at a 20° angle cranially. This gives better accessibility into the upper ankle joint. After the joint capsule has been penetrated, the needle drops into the joint line. The local anesthetic can be injected without increased pressure. Aspiration is vital prior to injection. The depth of insertion is 2 cm.

Risks

- The dorsalis pedis artery may be injured and the deep fibular nerve may be injured or anesthetized. This nerve runs parallel to the tendon of the extensor hallucis longus.
- **Strictly observe:** the injection must be performed medially to the tendon of the extensor hallucis longus.

Concomitant Therapies

- Anti-inflammatory support bandages, for example, Unna paste bandage
- Dynamic orthopedic ankle support, axial cushioning through buffer heels
- Iontophoresis
- TENS treatment

! ++
R once a week
PhysApps, Med, Orthotech

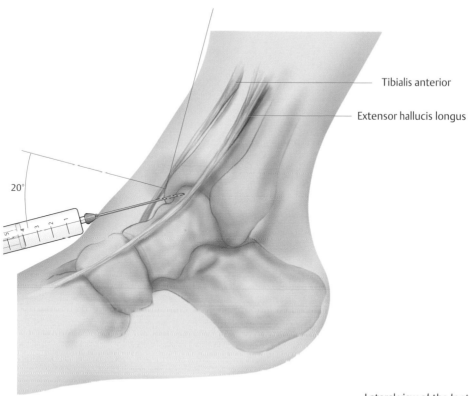

Tibialis anterior

Extensor hallucis longus

20°

Lateral view of the foot

Tibialis anterior

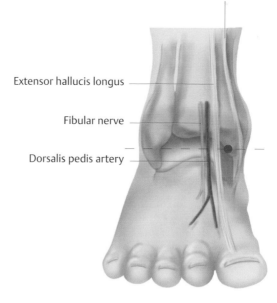

Extensor hallucis longus

Fibular nerve

Dorsalis pedis artery

Metatarsal Phalangeal Joint

Indications

- Arthritis
- Arthrosis of the metatarsal phalangeal joint
- Posttraumatic gout attack

Differential Diagnoses

- Sesamoiditis
- Bursitis at the first metatarsal head

Material

- Local anesthetic: 1–2 mL
- Needle: 0.4 × 20 mm

Technique

- The patient is in the supine position, the knee is in 45° flexion, and the foot is placed flat on the treatment surface. With use of the thumb nail, the joint line is an easily palpable depression. To confirm the palpation, the patient's big toe is passively moved into dorsal and plantar flexion. The joint line is marked and the free hand puts light distraction on the patient's big toe.
- The needle is inserted vertically. After the joint capsule has been penetrated, the joint cartilage is reached quickly; therefore, the needle must be advanced cautiously with light pressure on the plunger. The local anesthetic can be injected effortlessly if the needle tip is positioned correctly in the joint capsule.

Risks

- Intracapsular injection; here, the local anesthetic can only be injected with noticeable effort.

Concomitant Therapies

- Shoe adjustment
- Orthotics especially fitted for the metatarsal phalangeal joint, hallux rigidus roll
- Topical ant-inflammatory application
- Traction mobilization of the basal joint

! ++
Orthotech, MM

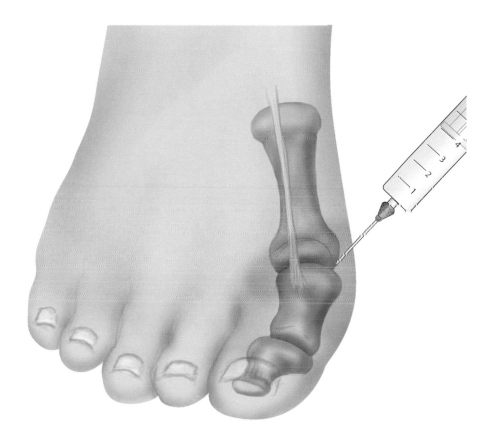

8 Myofascial Pain Syndromes

■ Frontoparietal Dysfunction Syndromes

Indications

- Mandibular joint dysfunctions
- Pressure sensitivity of the masticatory muscles
- Mandibular joint clicking
- Restricted mouth opening

Differential Diagnoses

- Arthritis of the mandibular joint
- Inflammation of dental roots
- Osseous processes of the jaw
- Parotitis

Material

- Local anesthetic: 3 mL
- Needle: 0.4 × 20 mm

Technique

- Depending on pain projection, the injectable is administered to myofascial trigger points of a superficial or a deep layer of the masseter.
- If pain is present in the area of the cheeks, paranasal sinuses, and upper jaw, the myofascial trigger point is found in the cranial superficial layer of the masseter. If pain extends toward the lower molars and the lower jaw, the injection sites are located in the deep layers of the central muscle belly of the masseter. Pain projected to the temples, above the eyebrow, and into the lower jaw originates in trigger points located in superficial caudal aspects of the masseter. Pain projected to the preauricular aspect of the ear and to the jaw angle is connected to a trigger point of the deep layer of the masseter, near its attachment to the zygomatic arch.
- At the proximal trigger points, the needle is inserted vertically 1 cm into the anterior and central aspect of the zygomatic arch. The injection sites are 1 cm apart. Each site receives 0.5–1 mL of a local anesthetic.
- Two injections are given to the central muscle belly of the masseter. The injection sites are located 2 cm apart. The needle is inserted vertically 1 cm and 1 mL of a local anesthetic is administered at each site while the muscle is completely tightened by the patient clenching the teeth.
- In distal myogelosis, the jaw angle is located. The two injection sites are found 2 cm apart, anterior to the jaw angle and 1 cm cranially. The needle is inserted vertically 0.5 cm and 1 mL of a local anesthetic is injected at both sites.
- If pain is most intense in front of the auricle, the zygomatic arch is located; while opening and closing the patient's mouth, the physician palpates the mandibular joint. Anterior to the mandibular joint, at the inferior edge of the zygomatic arch, the needle is inserted vertically 1.5 cm and 1.5 mL of a local anesthetic is injected.

Risks

- Intra-articular injection into the mandibular joint; therefore, locating the joint by opening and closing the patient's mouth prior to injection is imperative. If the needle is advanced excessively, the facial nerve may be anesthetized and the maxillary artery injured. The course of the maxillary artery varies considerably. Aspiration prior to injection is mandatory.

Concomitant Therapies

- Postisometric relaxation of the masseter
- Treatment of the mandibular joint using manual therapy
- Orthodontic treatment
- Cryogenic friction massage and self-mobilization

! +++
R 3 times a week, up to 6 weeks
PIR, MM, PhysApps, Orthodont

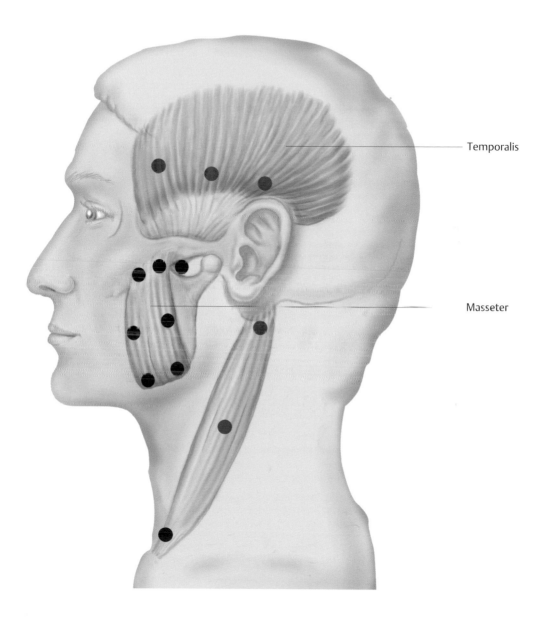

Temporalis

Masseter

● Primarily indicated injection points

● Complementary point

■ Occipitocervical Dysfunction Syndromes

Indications

- Dysfunctions accompanied by referred frontal and occipital headache

Differential Diagnoses

- Glaucoma
- Occipital neuralgia
- Tension headache

Material

- Local anesthetic: 4 mL
- Needle: 0.4 × 40 mm

Technique

- Supraorbitally, in a depression following the course of the eyebrow, the needle is inserted vertically and a quaddle is set containing 0.1 mL of a local anesthetic. The needle is advanced 4–5 mm and 0.4 mL of the local anesthetic is applied. The procedure is repeated on the other side.
- The occipitalis muscle is then located on the occiput. It is found occipitolateral, at the level of the superior auricular border. A rough, extremely pressure sensitive trigger point can be palpated at this site. The needle is inserted vertically and a quaddle is set containing 0.1 mL of a local anesthetic. The needle is then advanced up to the periosteum and after it has been retracted slightly, 0.4 mL of the injectable is administered. The same procedure is repeated on the occipitalis on the opposite side.

Risks

- None
- Intraperiosteal and subperiosteal injections are extremely painful and must be avoided.

Concomitant Therapies

- Biofeedback training
- Progressive relaxation techniques
- Mobilizing treatments and transverse friction using manual therapy

---

! ++
R 2 times a week, up to 6 weeks
PIR, MM, Med

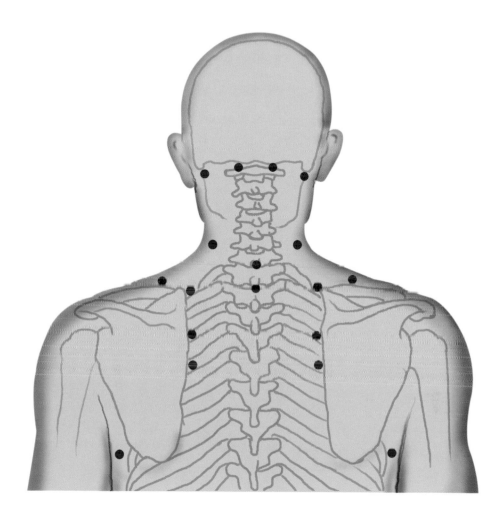

● Primarily indicated injection points

● Complementary point

Further Reading

Auberger HG et al. Praktische Lokalanästhesie. 4. Aufl. Stuttgart: Thieme; 1982

Augustin M et al. Praxisleitfaden Naturheilkunde. 2. Aufl. Neckarsulm: Jungjohann; 1994

Albrecht R et al. Regionalanästhesie. 2. Aufl. Stuttgart: Gustav Fischer; 1985

Bell WE. Orofacial Pains – Differential Diagnosis. Ed. 2. Chicago: Year Book Medical Publishers; 1979: 85, 200–203; Figs. 7–8, 7–9

Covino BG et al. Local Anaesthetics. Mechanisms of Action an clinical Use. New York: Grune & Stratton; 1976

Cyriax J. Textbook of Orthopaedic Medicine. Ed. 8, Vol. 2: Treatment by Manipulation, Massage and Injection. Baltimore: Williams & Wilkins; 1971

de Jong RH. Local Anaesthetic. Springfield: Illinois; 1977

de Jong RH. Defining Pain Terms. JAMA 1980; 244: 143

Dexter JR, Simons DG. Local Twitch Response in human Muscle evoked by Palpation and Needle Penetration or a Trigger Point. Arch Phys Med Rehabil 1982; 62: 521

Dosch P, Dosch M. Manual of Neural Therapy According to Huneke. 2nd ed. Stuttgart: Thieme; 2006

Dosch MP. Atlas of Neural Therapy. With Local Anesthetics. 2nd ed. Stuttgart: Thieme; 2003

Eder M. Herdgeschehen – Komplexgeschehen. Heidelberg: Haug; 1977

Eder M. Pathogenese und Klinik pseudoradikulärer Schmerzbilder. Man Med 1981; 54

Gabka J. Injektions- und Infusionstechniken. Praxis, Komplikationen und forensische Konsequenzen. 4. Aufl. Berlin: de Gruyter; 1988

Gabka J. Medizinische Geräte und Behältnisse für Transfusion, Infusion und Injektion. Din e. V. 2001

Greene CS. Myofascial Pain-Dysfunction Syndrome; nonsurgical Treatment. In: Sarnat BG, Laskin DM, eds. The temporomandibular Joint. 3. Aufl. Charles C. Thomas, Springfield: Illinois; 1980

Grill F. Die Behandlung von Schmerzsyndromen der Orthopädie mit Akupunktur. Handbuch der Akupunktur und Aurikulotherapie. Heidelberg: Haug; 1977

Gross D. Therapeutische Lokalanästhesie. 3. Aufl. Stuttgart: Hippokrates; 1985

Grosshandler S, Burney R. The myofascial Syndrome. NC Med J 1979; 40: 562–565

Gunn CC, Milbrandt WE. Tenderness at Motor Points. J Bone Joint Surg 1976; 58–A: 815–825

Head H. Die Sensibilitätsstörungen der Haut bei Viszeralerkrankungen. Berlin: Hirschwald; 1898

Hecker H-U, Steveling A, Peuker E, Kastner J, Liebchen K. Color Atlas of Acupuncture. Body Points – Ear Points – Trigger Points. 2nd ed. Stuttgart: Thieme; 2008

Hecker H-U. Practice of Acupuncture. Point Location – Treatment Options – TCM Basics. Stuttgart: Thieme 2004

Hempen C-H, Wortman V. Pocket Atlas of Acupuncture. Stuttgart: Thieme; 2005

Hilsche H. Beeinflußbarkeit von Erkrankungen, besonders des Bewegungsapparates, mittels segmental applizierter Lokaltherapie. In: Clud K, Hrsg. Perkutane Rheumatherapie. Frankfurt: Pharma Medical; 1980

Hirschberg GG, Froetscher I, Naeim F. Iliolumbar Syndrome as a common Cause of low Back Pain: Diagnosis and Prognosis. Arch Phys Med Rehabil 1979; 60: 415–419

Hunnecke W. Impletol Therapie. Stuttgart: Hippokrates; 1952

Ignelzi RJ, Atkinson JH. Pain and its Modulation. Part 2 – efferent Mechanisms. Neurosurgery 1980; 6: 584–590

Ingbar SH, Woeber KA. Diseases of the Thyroid, Chapter 335. In: Isselbacher KJ, Adams RD, Braunwald E et al., eds. Principles of internal Medicine. 9. Aufl. New York: McGraw-Hill Book Company; 1980: 1696, 1698–1699, 1701–1703, 1711

Kesson M, Atkins E, Davies I. Injektionen in Gelenke, Sehnen und Muskel. Praktische Injektionstechniken und Indikationen. 2. Aufl. Bern: Huber; 2008

Killian H. Lokalanästhesie und Lokalanästhetika. 2. Aufl. Stuttgart: Thieme; 1973

Kotani H, Kawazoe Y, Hamada T et al. Quantitative electromyographic Diagnosis of myofascial Pain-Dysfunction Syndrome. J Prosthet Dent 1980; 43: 450–456

Lewit K. Muskelfaszilitations- und Inhibitionstechniken in der Manuellen Medizin. Teil II: Postisometrische Muskelrelaxation. Man Med 1981; 19: 12–22

McCarty W. Diagnosis and Treatment of internal Derangements of the articular Disc and mandibular Condyle, Chapter 8. In: Solberg WK, Clark GT, eds. Temporomandibular Joint Problems. Chicago: Quintessence Publishing; 1980: 145–168

Macdonald jr. A. Abnormally tender Muscle Regions and associated painful Movements. Pain 1980; 8: 197–205

McNeill C, Danzig WM, Farrar WB et al. Craniomandibular (TMI) Disorders – the State of the Art. J Prosthet Dent 1980; 44: 434–437

Mahan PE. Differential Diagnosis of craniofacial Pain and Dysfunction. Alpha Omega 1976; 69: 42–49

Maigne R. Low Back Pain of thoracolumbar Origin. Arch Phys Med Rehabil 1980; 61: 389–395

Meier G, Buettner J. Peripheral Regional Anesthesia. An Atlas of Anatomy and Techniques. 2nd ed. Stuttgart: Thieme; 2007

Melzack R, Jeans ME, Stratford JG et al. Ice Massage and transcutaneous electrical Stimulation: Comparison of Treatment for low Back Pain. Pain 1980; 9: 209–217

Mercuri LG, Olson RE, Laskin DM. The Specificity of Response to experimental Stress in Patients with myofascial Pain Dysfunction Syndrome. J Dent Res 1979; 58: 1866–1871

Meyer JH. Die Pharmakologie, Toxikologie und klinische Anwendung lang wirkender Lokalanästhetika. Stuttgart: Thieme; 1977

Mikhail M, Rosen H. History and Etiology of myofascial Pain-Dysfunction Syndrome. J Prosthet Dent 1980; 44: 438–444

Moore DC. Regionalblock. 4. Aufl. Springfield: Illinois; 1965

Morgan jr. GJ. Panniculitis and erythema Nodosum, Chapter 75. In: Kelley WN, Harris ED, Ruddy S et al. Textbook of Rheumatology. Vol. 2. Philadelphia: WB Saunders; 1981: 1203–1207

Niesel HC. Regionalanästhesie. Stuttgart: Gustav Fischer; 1981

Nolte H. Die Technik der Lokalanästhesie. Berlin: Springer; 1966

Reichert B, Palpation Techniques. Stuttgart: Thieme; 2010

Reynolds MD. Myofascial Trigger Point Syndromes in the Practice of Rheumatology. Arch Phys Med Rehabil 1981; 62: 111–114, Tables 1 and 2

Reynolds MD. The Development of the Concept of Fibrositis. J Hist Med Allied Science 1983: 103–118

Richter P, Hebgen E. Trigger Points and Muscle Chains in Osteopathy. Stuttgart: Thieme; 2008

Rubin D. An Approach to the Management of myofascial Trigger Point Syndromes. Arch Phys Med Rehabil 1981; 62: 107–110

Sherman RA. Published Treatments of Phantom Limb Pain. Am J Phys Med 1980; 59: 232–244

Simons DG, Travell JG. The Latissimus Dorsi Syndrome: a Source of mid-Back Pain. Arch Phys Med Rehabil 1976; 57: 561

Simons DG, Travell J. Common myofascial Origins of low Back Pain. Postgrad Med 1983; 73: 66–108

Smythe HA. Fibrositis and other diffuse musculoskeletal Syndromes. In: Kelley WN, Harris jr. ED, Ruddy S et al., eds. Textbook of Rheumatology, Vol. 1. Philadelphia: WB Saunders; 1981: 489

Theodoridis T, Kraemer J. Spinal Injection Techniques. Stuttgart: Thieme; 2009

Tilscher H et al. Lehrbuch der Reflextherapie. Stuttgart: Hippokrates; 1986

Travell J. Identification of myofascial Trigger Point Syndromes: a Case of atypical facial Neuralgia. Arch Phys Med Rehabil 1981; 62: 100–106

Wyant GM. Chronic Pain Syndromes and their Treatment. II: Trigger Points. Can Anaesth Soc J 1979; 26: 216–219, Patients 1 and 2

Yagiela JA, Benoit PW, Buoncristiani RD et al. Comparison of myotoxic Effects of Lidocaine with Epinephrine in Rats and Humans. Anesth Analg 1981; 60: 471–480

Zimmermann M. Physiologiemechanismen von Schmerzen und Schmerztherapie. Triangel 1981; 20: 1–2

Index

Page numbers in *italics* refer to illustrations